The Managed Health Care Handbook Series

Managed Care
What It Is and How It Works
Second Edition

The Managed Health Care Handbook Series

The Managed Health Care Handbook, Fourth Edition
Peter R. Kongstvedt

Essentials of Managed Health Care, Fourth Edition
Peter R. Kongstvedt

Best Practices in Medical Management
Peter R. Kongstvedt, David W. Plocher

Managed Care: What It Is and How It Works, Second Edition
Peter R. Kongstvedt

Managed Care
What It Is and How It Works
Second Edition

Peter R. Kongstvedt, MD
Cap Gemini Ernst & Young
McLean, VA

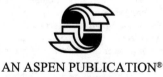

AN ASPEN PUBLICATION®
Aspen Publishers, Inc.
Gaithersburg, Maryland
2002

Library of Congress Cataloging-in-Publication Data

Kongstvedt, Peter R. (Peter Reid)
Managed care: what it is and how it works/Peter R. Kongstvedt.—2nd ed.
p. cm. (The managed health care handbook series)
Much of the material found in this book has been distilled from the parent text:
The managed health care handbook, 4th ed.
Includes bibliographical references and index.
ISBN 0-8342-2089-X
1. Managed care plans (Medical care)—United States. I. Managed health care
handbook. II. Title. III. Series.
RA413.5.U5 K655 2002
362.1'04258'0973—dc21
2001055993

Copyright © 2002 by Aspen Publishers, Inc.
A Wolters Kluwer Company
www.aspenpublishers.com
All rights reserved.

Orders: (800) 638-8437
Customer Service: (800) 234-1660

About Aspen Publishers • For more than 40 years, Aspen has been a leading professional publisher in a variety of disciplines. Aspen's vast information resources are available in both print and electronic formats. We are committed to providing the highest quality information available in the most appropriate format for our customers. Visit Aspen's Internet site for more information resources, directories, articles, and a searchable version of Aspen's full catalog, including the most recent publications: **www.aspenpublishers.com**
Aspen Publishers, Inc. • The hallmark of quality in publishing
Member of the worldwide Wolters Kluwer group

Editorial Services: Joan Sesma
Library of Congress Catalog Card Number: 2001055993
ISBN: 0-8342-2089-X

Printed in the United States of America

1 2 3 4 5

Contents

Preface

Since the first edition of *Managed Care: What It Is and How It Works* was published, managed care has evolved at a rapid pace, and all expectations are that it will continue to evolve. It is almost a certainty that new approaches to managing cost, quality, and access will be developed, some of these will fail, while others will succeed and lead to still more changes. Indeed, the health care industry can be described as caught in "permanent white water." For some, this means heavy rapids; for others, it means Niagara Falls. Now more than ever, individuals who are involved with the management of health care need to be quick and adaptive. As the best river guides know, rafters should not fight the current but use it to their advantage.

Health care costs have risen at variable rates. The shocking increases experienced in the early 1990s slowed in the mid-1990s but have begun to appear again at the turn of the 21st century. Managed care has been effective in holding down the rate of rise, but many of the fundamental reasons for increased health care costs remain today. These include the following:

- rapidly developing (and usually expensive) medical technology

- drug therapy advances and rising prescription drug prices
- shifting demographics, especially the "aging" of the population
- high (and not unreasonable) expectations for a long and healthy life
- greater control of health care by consumers and associated greater demands upon the health care system
- the litigiousness of our society, which leads physicians to practice defensive medicine
- high administrative costs related to the care that is delivered
- inefficient or poor quality care rendered by some providers (professional and institutional)
- high incomes for some types of providers (regardless of efficiency or quality)
- high cost of compliance with government mandates
- decreased levels of public dollars to pay for entitlement program health care
- cost shifting by providers to pay for health care rendered to patients who either cannot pay or are covered by systems that do not pay the full cost of care

The continued expansion of knowledge and increased complexity in the managed care industry make it necessary to address new issues as well as revise and update earlier discussions of better known issues. Of equal importance, other sectors of the health care system are changing as well, often as a response to changes in managed care. For example, physicians do not exhibit the same types of practice behaviors that were prevalent a decade ago, hospital usage rates have declined across the nation (though not to uniform levels), and new diagnostic and therapeutic interventions have appeared. Changes in the other health care sectors in turn are causing further changes in managed care, keeping the health care system in a state of turbulence.

Besides continuing to be turbulent, the health care system is becoming more complex—and at an ever faster though unsteady pace. As a result, future states of the system are impossible to predict exactly. Readers of *Managed Care: What It Is and How It Works* should therefore recognize the true vitality of managed care and not fall into the trap of thinking that it offers only one way to do something. Yet, in a field this complex, it is essential to begin with basic descriptions of the most prominent topics. This book does exactly that, as indicated by the following chapter summaries.

Chapter 1 focuses on the history and evolution of managed care. It provides the background necessary for readers to understand the nature of managed care as it exists today.

Chapter 2 describes the main types of managed care organizations (MCO) and integrated health care delivery systems. It also reviews the basic governance and management structure of health plans.

Chapter 3 is an overview of the health care delivery system. It describes the basic provider sectors—primary care physicians, specialty physicians, and hospitals and other health care institutions—and the way that managed care works within them. It also covers the topics of network development, network management, and reimbursement.

Chapter 4 explains how managed care actually manages health care. The basics components of medical management include medical-surgical utilization management (including authorization systems), case and disease management, management of pharmaceutical services, and quality management. Managed care is not simply about approving or denying payment for a health care service or contracting for favorable pricing; it is also about changing the way that health care is delivered.

Chapter 5 presents an account of the nonmedical operations of MCOs. The functions described include the claims processing, information management, marketing and sales, member services, underwriting, and financial management. These are the foundational functions of any health plan and they must operate properly for the plan to succeed.

Chapter 6 describes the Medicare and Medicaid programs and their increasing use of managed care to control costs, enhance the coordination of care, and improve its quality. It defines some of the differences between the two programs and indicates some of the ways that MCOs undertaking to serve Medicare and Medicaid populations must modify their operations to meet the programs' special requirements.

Chapter 7 focuses on the regulation of managed care. States continue to play a dominant role in the regulation of health plans, and a section on state requirements leads the chapter. Following that section is a discussion of a new federal law, the Health Insurance Portability and Accountability Act of 1996 (HIPAA), which has hugely important implications for electronic interactions, privacy, and information security in all parts of the health care industry. Another important federal law, the Employee Retirement Income Security Act (ERISA), which regulates self-funded health benefits plans, is briefly discussed. Lastly, the chapter describes the accreditation of MCOs.

The *Epilogue* speculates on the future of managed care and offers a tool—a list of factors likely to influence the health care system—to help readers reach their own conclusions on where managed care is headed.

The book ends with a comprehensive glossary that provides definitions of terms commonly used in the managed care industry.

Much of the material found in this book has been distilled from the parent text of this series: *The Managed Health Care Handbook*. Interested readers wanting additional information about most aspects of managed care are advised to consult this comprehensive reference work, whose fourth edition was published by Aspen Publishers in 2000.

The main goal of this book is very simple—to provide its readers with a solid understanding of how managed care actually works. If it succeeds in doing that, then some who are reading these words right now will be in a position to better contribute to the future evolution of this dynamic industry, thereby benefiting us all.

CHAPTER 1

The Origins of Managed Care

LEARNING OBJECTIVES

- Understand how managed care came into being
- Understand the forces that have shaped managed care in the past
- Understand the major obstacles to managed care historically
- Understand the major forces shaping managed care today

MANAGED CARE: THE EARLY YEARS (PRE–1970)

Sometimes cited as the first example of a health maintenance organization (HMO), the Western Clinic in Tacoma, Washington began in 1910 to offer, exclusively through its own providers, a broad range of medical services in return for a premium payment of $0.50 per member per month. The program was available to lumber mill owners and their employ-

---

Source: Adapted from P.D. Fox, An Overview of Managed care, in *The Managed Health Care Handbook,* 4th ed., P.R. Kongstvedt, ed., pp. 3–16, © 2000, Aspen Publishers, Inc.

ees, and it served to ensure a flow of patients and revenues for the clinic. A similar program that was later developed in Tacoma expanded to 20 sites in Oregon and Washington.

In 1929, Dr. Michael Shadid established a rural farmers' cooperative health plan in Elk City, Oklahoma. Participating farmers purchased shares for $50 each to raise capital for a new hospital; in return, they received medical care at a discount. Because of the medical community's opposition to this new concept, Shadid lost his membership in the county medical society and was threatened with suspension of his license to practice medicine. Some 20 years later, however, he was vindicated through an out-of-court settlement in his favor of an antitrust suit against the county and state medical societies. In 1934, the Farmers Union assumed control of both the hospital and the health plan.

As Starr noted,* health insurance itself is of relatively recent origin. In 1929, Baylor Hospital in Texas agreed to provide some 1,500 teachers with prepaid care at its hospital, an arrangement that represented the origins of Blue Cross. The program was subsequently expanded to include other employers and hospitals, initially through single hospital plans. Starting in 1939, a number of state medical societies, such as that in California, created Blue Shield plans to cover physician services. At the time, commercial health insurance was not a factor.

The formation of the various Blue Cross and Blue Shield plans, as well as the beginning of many HMOs, in the midst of the Great Depression came about, not because consumers

*P. Starr, *The Social Transformation of American Medicine* (New York: Basic Books, 1982).

were demanding insurance against the risk of medical expenses or because nonphysician entrepreneurs were seeking to establish a business, but rather because providers wanted to maintain and enhance patient revenues. Many of these developments were threatening to organized medicine. In 1932, the American Medical Association (AMA) adopted a strong position against prepaid group practices, favoring instead indemnity type insurance that protects the policyholder from expenses by reimbursment. The AMA took this stance in response to the prepaid group practices in existence at the time (although few in number) and to the findings in 1932 of the Committee on the Cost of Medical Care—a highly visible private group of leaders from medicine, dentistry, public health, consumers, and so forth—that recommended the expansion of group practice as an efficient health care delivery system. The AMA's opposition set the tone for continued state and local medical society resistance to prepaid group practice at the state and local medical society levels.

The period immediately surrounding World War II saw the formation of several HMOs, some of which remain prominent today. They represent a diversity of origins, as the initial impetus came variously from employers seeking benefits for their employees, providers seeking patient revenues, consumers seeking access to improved and affordable health care, and even a housing lending agency seeking a reduction in the number of foreclosures. The following are examples of early HMOs:

- The Kaiser Foundation Health Plans were started in 1937 by Dr. Sidney Garfield at the request of the Kaiser construction company. The purpose was to finance medical care for workers who were building an aqueduct in the southern California desert to transport water from the Colorado River to Los Angeles and, subsequently, for workers who were constructing the Grand Coulee Dam in Washington State. A similar program was established in 1942 at Kaiser shipbuilding plants in the San Francisco Bay area.

- In 1937, the Home Owner's Loan Corporation organized the Group Health Association (GHA) in Washington, D.C. to reduce the number of mortgage defaults by families that had large medical expenses. It was a nonprofit consumer cooperative, with the board of directors elected periodically by the enrollees. The District of Columbia Medical Society opposed the formation of GHA, seeking to restrict hospital admitting privileges for GHA physicians and threatening to expel those physicians from the medical society. A bitter antitrust battle ensued that culminated in the U.S. Supreme Court's ruling in favor of GHA. In 1994, GHA was facing insolvency despite an enrollment of some 128,000 members. Humana Health Plans, a for-profit, publicly traded corporation, acquired GHA but has since disbanded it. The membership now belongs to the Kaiser Foundation Health Plan of the Mid-Atlantic.
- In 1944, in response to the needs of New York City seeking coverage for its employees, the Health Insurance Plan (HIP) of Greater New York was formed.
- In 1947, consumers in Seattle organized 400 families, who contributed $100 each, to form the Group Health Cooperative of Puget Sound. Predictably, the Kings County Medical Society opposed the cooperative.

These pioneer prepaid group practices encountered varying degrees of opposition from local medical societies.

Only in later years did nonprovider entrepreneurs form for-profit HMOs in significant numbers. The early independent practice association (IPA) model HMOs, which contract with physicians in independent fee-for-service practice, were developed as a way of competing with group practice–based HMOs. The basic structure was created in 1954, when the San Joaquin County Medical Society in California formed the San Joaquin Medical Foundation in response to competition from the Kaiser Foundation Health Plans. The San Joaquin Medical Foundation established a relative value fee schedule for paying physicians, heard grievances against physicians, and monitored the quality of health care. It received a license from the state to accept a set monthly fee (i.e., capitation payment) to provide for each person enrolled in the plan all the health care services that he or she needed, making it the first IPA model HMO.

THE ADOLESCENT YEARS OF MANAGED CARE: 1970–1985

Through the 1960s and into the early 1970s, HMOs played only a modest role in the financing and delivery of health care. Although they were a significant presence in a few communities, such as the Seattle area and parts of California, the total number of HMOs nationwide in 1970 fell somewhere in the 30s, the exact number depending on the definition used. The period since the early 1970s has seen vastly accelerated developments that are still unfolding.

The major boost to the HMO movement during this period was the enactment in 1973 of the federal Health Maintenance Organization Act. That act authorized start-up funding and, more important, ensured access to the employer-based health insurance market. The act evolved from discussions that Dr. Paul Ellwood had in 1970 with the officials of the U.S. Department of Health, Education and Welfare (which later became the U.S. Department of Health and Human Services). Ellwood had participated in designing the Health Planning Act of 1966 during the presidency of Lyndon Johnson.

Ellwood, sometimes referred to as the father of the modern HMO movement, was asked in the early years of the Nixon Administration to devise ways of constraining the increases in the Medicare budget. His conversations with federal officials lead to a proposal to reimburse HMOs for Medicare beneficiaries' health care through a capitation system (a proposal that was not enacted until 1982) and laid the groundwork for what became the HMO Act of 1973. The emphasis on HMOs at this time reflected the perspective that the fee-for-service system, by rewarding physicians for providing more services rather than for providing appropriate services, incorporated the wrong incentives. Also, the term *health maintenance organization* was coined then as a substitute for *prepaid group practice,* principally because it had greater public appeal.

The main features of the HMO Act were these:

- It made grants and loans available for the planning and start-up phases of new HMOs as well as for service area expansions for existing HMOs.

- It overrode state laws that restricted the development of HMOs if the HMOs met federal requirements for certification.
- Most important of all, it required employers with 25 or more employees that offered indemnity coverage also to offer two federally certified HMO options if the plans made a formal request. For workers under collective bargaining agreements, the union had to agree to the offering. Many HMOs were reluctant to exercise the mandate, fearing that making such a request would antagonize employers and cause them to discourage employees from enrolling. However, many other HMOs used the dual choice provision to at least advertise themselves to employer groups.

The statute also established a process under which HMOs could elect to obtain federal certification. Unlike state licensure, which is mandatory, federal certification has always been at the discretion of the individual HMO. To obtain federal certification, HMOs had to satisfy a series of requirements, such as meeting minimum benefit package standards set forth in the act, demonstrating that their provider networks were adequate, having a quality assurance system in place, complying with standards of financial stability, and establishing an enrollee grievance system. Some states emulated these requirements and adopted them for all HMOs that were licensed in the state, regardless of federal certification status.

Plans that requested federal certification did so for four principal reasons. First, certification represented a "Seal of

Approval" that was helpful in marketing. Second, the required offering of HMO options ensured that HMOs that were federally certified would have access to the employer market. Third, the override of state laws—important in some states but not in others—applied only to federally qualified HMOs. Fourth, only those HMOs that obtained federal certification could receive the federal grants and loans that were available during the early years of the act. Federal certification is less important today than it was when managed care was in its infancy and HMOs were struggling for inclusion in employment-based health benefit programs, which account for most private insurance in the United States. As HMOs have matured in the marketplace and become mainstream, the advantages that federal certification lent are no longer necessary.

The HMO Act also contained provisions that some believed were retarding the growth of HMOs. The existence of these provisions stemmed from a compromise in Congress between two camps. One camp was interested principally in fostering competition in the health care marketplace by promoting plans that incorporated incentives for providers to control costs. The second camp, while perhaps sharing the objectives of the first, saw the HMO Act principally as a precursor to health care reform and sought a way to expand access to coverage for individuals who were without insurance or who had only limited benefits. Imposing requirements on HMOs but not on indemnity carriers, however, reduced the ability of HMOs to compete with the indemnity carriers. Requirements imposed solely on federally qualified HMOs included significant restrictions on how they created premium rates to charge to businesses and individuals; requiring HMOs to enroll any individual regardless of their health status; and a far richer benefits package than existed in the typical indemnity insurance plan.

Of particular note were requirements pertaining to the comprehensiveness of the benefits package as well as open enrollment and community rating. The open enrollment provision required that plans accept individuals and groups without regard to their health status. The provision for community rating of premiums, which mandated that HMOs seek the same fees per member for all members in the plan limited the ability of HMOs to tie premium levels to the health status of the individual enrollee or employer group. Both provisions represented laudable public policy goals; the problem was that, as noted previously, they had the potential for making federally certified HMOs noncompetitive because the same requirements did not apply to the traditional insurance plans against which they competed. The enactment of amendments to the HMO Act in the late 1970s largely corrected this situation by reducing some of the more onerous requirements. The federal dual choice provisions were "sunsetted" (allowed to expire) in 1995 and are no longer in effect

The slowness of the federal government in issuing the regulations implementing the act also delayed HMO development. Employers knew that they would have to contract with federally certified plans. Even those that supported the mandate had to wait until the government determined which plans would be qualified and established the processes for implementing the dual choice provisions. In 1977, however, at the beginning of the Carter administration, issuance of the regulations became a priority and rapid growth ensued.

Politically, several aspects of this history are noteworthy. For example, although differences arose on specifics, congressional support for legislation promoting HMO development came from both political parties. Also, there was no widespread state opposition to the federal override of restrictive state laws. In addition, most employers did not actively oppose the dual choice requirements, although many disliked being required to contract with HMOs by the federal government. Perhaps most interesting of all has been the generally positive interaction between the public sector and the private sector, with government fostering HMO development both through its regulatory processes and its purchase of health care coverage under its employee benefits programs.

Among the other managed care developments that took place during the 1970s and early 1980s was the creation of the preferred provider organization (PPO), a plan that contracts with a limited number of independent providers to obtain services for its members at a discount. It is generally believed that the PPO originated in Denver, where in the early 1970s Samuel Jenkins, a vice president of the benefits consulting firm of the Martin E. Segal Company, negotiated discounts with hospitals on behalf of the company's Taft-Hartley trust fund clients. Utilization review also evolved outside the HMO setting between 1970 and 1985, although it has earlier origins:

- In 1959, Blue Cross of Western Pennsylvania, the Allegheny County Medical Society Foundation, and the Hospital Council of Western Pennsylvania performed retrospective analyses of hospital claims to identify utilization that was significantly above average.

- Around 1970, California's Medicaid program began to require preadmission authorization for routine hospitalizations and concurrent review in conjunction with medical care foundations in the state, starting with the Sacramento Foundation for Medical Care. Such foundations were not-for-profit organizations, usually created by local organized medicine or medical societies, for purposes of conducting utilization review and later, to create independent practice association types of HMOs.
- The 1972 Social Security Amendments authorized the federal Professional Standards Review Organization (PSRO) program to review the appropriateness of care provided to Medicare and Medicaid beneficiaries. Although its effectiveness has been debated, the PSRO program established an organizational infrastructure and data capacity upon which both the public and private sectors could rely.
- In the 1970s, a handful of large corporations initiated programs for preauthorization and concurrent review for inpatient care.

Developments in indemnity insurance, mostly during the 1980s, included (1) encouraging persons with conventional insurance to obtain second opinions before undergoing elective surgery and (2) adopting "large case management" (i.e., the coordination of services for persons with conditions that require expensive medical care, such as selected accident patients, cancer patients, and very low birthweight infants). Also during the 1980s, worksite wellness programs became more prevalent as employers, in varying degrees and in varying ways, instituted such programs as the following:

- screening (e.g., for hypertension and diabetes)
- health risk appraisal
- exercise promotion (whether by providing access to gyms, conveniently located showers, or running paths or by simply providing information)
- stress reduction
- classes (e.g., smoking cessation, weight lifting)
- nutrition, including the serving of healthy food in the cafeteria
- weight loss
- mental health counseling

MANAGED CARE AS A MATURE CONCEPT: 1985–1995

The period between 1985 and 1995 saw a combination of innovation, maturation, and restructuring.

Innovation

In many communities, physicians and hospitals collaborated to form physician-hospital organizations (PHOs), principally as vehicles for contracting with managed care organizations. Typically, PHOs are corporations in which the physicians and the hospital each have the right to designate half the members of the board of directors. Most PHOs sought to enter into fee-for-service arrangements with HMOs and PPOs, although an increasing number accept full capitation risk. Full risk capitation, as discussed in Chapter 3, involves the PHO accepting a fixed amount of money per member per month for all health care expenses. However, with the failure of many such full risk arrangements in the years 1999 and 2000, acceptance of full risk capitation has sharply declined.

For several reasons, PHOs did not become important elements of the managed care environment. Their reimbursement systems, for example, did not support the primary managed care goals of cost containment and efficient care. The typical PHO allowed all physicians with admitting privileges at the hospital to participate in the plan rather than selecting the more efficient ones, and it also required physicians to use the hospital for outpatient services (e.g., laboratory tests) that might have been available at lower cost elsewhere, hurting its price competitiveness. Finally, some PHOs were poorly organized, had inadequate information systems, operated under inexperienced management, or lacked the necessary capital for investment. In the end, PHOs with these kinds of problems were not able to sustain the financial risks.

The development of carve-out companies—organizations that have specialized provider networks that offer specific services, such as mental health care, management of a particular disease (e.g., congestive heart failure, diabetes), chiropractic treatment, and dental services—occurred during this period. The carve-out companies market their services primarily to HMOs and large self-insured employers. Similar in concept are groups of specialists, such as ophthalmologists and radiologists, who accept capitation risk for their services (sometimes referred to as subcapitation) through contracts with health plans and employer groups.

Advances in computer technology have made other innovations possible. Vastly improved computer programs, marketed by private firms or developed by managed care plans for internal use, can generate statistical profiles of the services rendered by physicians. These profiles serve not only as a means to assess the efficiency and the quality of the care that each physician provides but also as a basis for the adjustment of payment levels to providers who are paid under capitation or risk-sharing arrangements that reflect the severity of illness among each provider's patient group.

Computer technology is responsible for a virtual revolution in the processing of medical and drug claims. The increasingly widespread use of electronic processing rather than paper submission and manual entry has dramatically lowered administrative costs and broadened access to far superior information; when dispensing a prescription, for example, the pharmacist can now receive information about potential adverse effects and interactions. Management information systems can be expected to improve in the next few years as providers, almost universally, submit claims electronically. Requirements under the Health Insurance Portability and Accountability Act of 1996 (HIPAA) for administrative simplification will tremendously accelerate the movement toward inexpensive electronic interchange for the basic transactions in managed care, including

- claims
- claims status
- authorizations
- eligibility checking
- payment

Maturation

Managed care's maturation is evident from several vantage points. One is the enormous growth in MCO enrollment through the 1990s followed by a slight decline (Figure 1–1). Another is the nature of managed care enrollment by Medicare and Medicaid (Figures 1–2 and 1–3).

In the 1990s, many HMOs regarded their participation with the Medicare+Choice program as an essential part of their business strategy. As illustrated in Figure 1–2, enrollment in Medicare+Choice HMOs peaked in 2000, and now appears to be in decline.

The interest of health plans in contracting with Medicare arose from the belief that doing so could be profitable; that employers want HMO options for retirees; and that a plan could have a competitive advantage in negotiating reimbursement arrangements with its participating providers if those providers receive a high proportion of their income from the plan. The recent decline in HMOs with capitation contracts with the Centers for Medicare & Medicaid Services* (CMS) results from changes in the Balanced Budget Act of 1997, which reduced payment levels and imposed new administrative burdens on managed care organizations that provide care for Medicare beneficiaries. The Balanced Budget Act also calls for adjustments in payment levels to reflect the relative

---

*As of July 1, 2001, the Health Care Financing Administration (HCFA) is now the Centers for Medicare & Medicaid Services (CMS) (http://www.cms.gov).

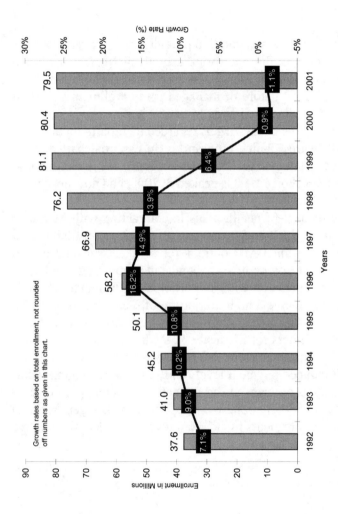

Figure 1–1 Total HMO enrollment and growth rate: January 1992 to January 2001. *Source:* Reprinted with permission from The InterStudy Competitive Edge: HMO Industry Report 11.2 (St. Paul, MN) © InterStudy.

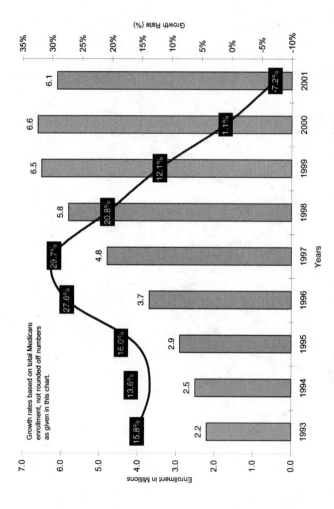

Figure 1–2 HMO Medicare enrollment and growth rate: January 1993 to January 2001. *Source:* Reprinted with permission from The InterStudy Competitive Edge: HMO Industry Report 11.2 (St. Paul, MN) © InterStudy.

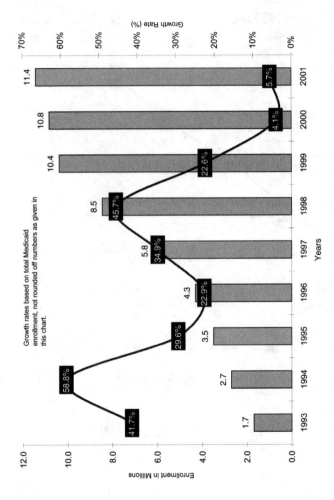

Figure 1–3 HMO Medicaid enrollment and growth rate: January 1993 to January 2001. *Source:* Reprinted with permission from The InterStudy Competitive Edge: HMO Industry Report 11.2 (St. Paul, MN) © InterStudy.

health status of enrollees; these adjustments are expected to further decrease payment to most health plans and, also, for at least several years, to make payment levels less predictable than before. Because of the reimbursement reductions, many plans began in January 2000 to increase premiums and reduce benefits; others dropped out of the program entirely. Despite a last minute effort by CMS in 2001 to provide slightly higher reimbursement rates to HMOs, the drop out rate of health plans continues.

State Medicaid programs, too, have turned to managed care, and are removing the fee-for-service option. As illustrated in Figure 1–3, growth in Medicaid managed care has been substantial and continues even today. Many beneficiaries not in a Medicaid HMO obtain care under less restrictive arrangements, mostly so-called primary care case management (PCCM) programs, in which beneficiaries choose a primary care physician who must approve referrals to specialists and other services. Under a PCCM program, providers are typically paid a fee for service, except that the primary care physician may receive a small monthly case management fee. Only a small percentage of beneficiaries who are eligible for both Medicare and Medicaid are in managed care because of various barriers in the Medicare program.

External quality oversight activities also indicate maturation. Launched by the HMO industry in 1979 to develop standards of quality and measure those standards on behalf of employers, the National Committee for Quality Assurance (NCQA) became independent in 1991 and began to accredit HMOs. Many employers are demanding or strongly encouraging NCQA accreditation of the HMOs with which they contract, and accreditation is coming to replace federal certification as the "seal of approval."

In addition, performance measurement systems (i.e., "report cards") are evolving, although they are now at an early stage. The most prominent is the Health Plan Employer Data and Information Set (HEDIS), which the NCQA developed at the behest of several large employers and health plans. The set of quality indicators is incomplete but will be improved over time. The performance measurement system currently focus too narrowly on what is easily measurable and lacks health outcome measures. As more and more of the insured lose access to traditional indemnity plans, the issue of HMO performance will become even more salient.

In the past, the focus of cost-management efforts was almost exclusively on inpatient hospital utilization. Practice patterns have changed dramatically in the last 20 years, however, and inpatient care has declined significantly. Although hospital admissions still receive considerable scrutiny, features of ambulatory care such as the use of prescription drugs, diagnostic tests, and visits to specialists are receiving greater attention.

Restructuring

Perhaps the most dramatic development in managed care is the restructuring that is occurring and that reflects the interplay between managed care and the health care delivery system. The distinctions among managed care organizations are blurring as each type begins to adopt features of the other types. For example, staff and group model HMOs, declining in number and facing limited capital and a need to expand into new territories, are taking on some of the characteristics of IPAs. Meanwhile, some IPAs have created staff model primary care centers while continuing to contract with physicians in independent practice for specialty services. Additionally, HMOs are offering preferred provider organization (PPO) and point-of-service plan products, and some PPOs are obtaining HMO licenses. In short, the managed care environment is becoming much more complicated.

Finally, consolidation is taking place among both health care plans and providers. Managed care plans with members in several states accounted for 60 percent of total enrollment nationally in 1994. Mergers are continuing to occur, as exemplified in the late 1990s by Aetna's acquisition of US HealthCare, NYLCare, and Prudential; CIGNA's purchase of HealthSource; acquisitions by WellPoint and by Anthem; and several of the Blue Cross and Blue Shield plan mergers.

MANAGED CARE IN RECENT TIMES

The economic boom of the mid- to late-1990s changed the dynamics in the managed care industry. As unemployment dropped below 4 percent, corporate profits became robust, and the economy grew, employers found it necessary to compete for employees. The anti–managed care rhetoric of political campaigns, combined with media "horror stories" about the unfortunate experiences of a few patients, helped fuel negative public sentiments about managed care. Despite generally positive perceptions of their own health plans (Figure 1–4), most consumers have negative perceptions about managed care in general (Figure 1–5).

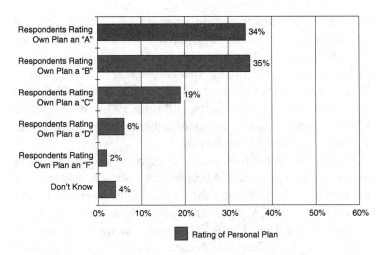

Figure 1–4 Respondents' general perceptions of their own health plans, December 2000. *Source:* Adapted with permission from *Health Care News,* Vol. 1, Issue 6, February 12, 2001, © Harris Interactive^SM.

As a result of these sentiments both among the public and among employers, many of the traditional techniques of managed care have undergone modification. For example, PPOs have grown in popularity despite their modestly higher costs. Furthermore, as utilization management becomes more sophisticated, there is more emphasis on management of high-cost chronic medical conditions and less on management of routine care

As mentioned in the Preface, benefits costs have begun to rise again for a number of reasons. At the same time, the economy has weakened. Consequently, consumers are facing

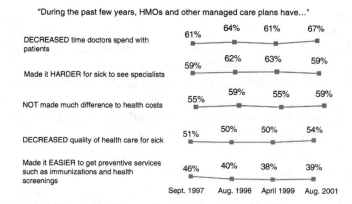

"During the past few years, HMOs and other managed care plans have…"

	Sept. 1997	Aug. 1998	April 1999	Aug. 2001
DECREASED time doctors spend with patients	61%	64%	61%	67%
Made it HARDER for sick to see specialists	59%	62%	63%	59%
NOT made much difference to health costs	55%	59%	55%	59%
DECREASED quality of health care for sick	51%	50%	50%	54%
Made it EASIER to get preventive services such as immunizations and health screenings	46%	40%	38%	39%

Figure 1–5 Outlook on managed care. *Source:* Reprinted with permission from *Kaiser Public Opinion Update,* August 2001, data from Kaiser Family Foundation/Harvard School of Public Health.

higher payroll deductions for health benefits coverage and changes in the benefits themselves. Copayments have been rising and in some cases are becoming more complex. For example, there has been a recent increase in three-tier pharmacy benefits—the lowest copayment is for generic drugs, a midlevel copayment is for brand-name drugs the managed care organization has placed in its formulary, and the highest copayment is for brand-name drugs not in the formulary. Ironically, shifting costs to consumers was the primary method of cost control available to indemnity insurance prior to the advent of managed care.

Consumer choice has also been increasing in importance, not only because of consumer demands but also because of the desire of employers to provide greater flexibility in the health benefit programs that they offer employees. With greater choice often come greater costs, however. Consumers find that in many cases they must choose between care that entails out-of-pocket costs and the managed care that is available to them. Beyond the issue of cost, managed care organizations are using technology such as the Internet to make it easier for consumers to choose physicians, benefits plans, and other features of health care plans.

CONCLUSION

Managed care is not disappearing. It is evolving, as it always has. It is not reasonable to believe that any health care system, including managed care, could remain fixed and unchanging. As the economic and clinical environment changes, so does managed care. HMOs have been highly successful, but are presently flat in enrollment as other forms of managed care plans such as PPOs grow. Managed care in Medicare was also highly successful, but has declined dramatically in recent years as it became financially non-viable. Further change in the ways managed care functions in our health care system is the only safe prediction one can make.

CHAPTER 2

Types of Managed Care Organizations and Their Structure

LEARNING OBJECTIVES

- Understand the basic managed care organization models
- Understand the differences between models
- Understand the principal services offered by managed care organizations
- Understand the primary structural components of managed care organizations

---

Defining the different types of managed care organizations (MCOs) is an ever-evolving challenge. Ten to fifteen years ago, it was relatively easy to distinguish among different types of MCOs. Health maintenance organizations (HMOs), preferred provider organizations (PPOs), and the more recent point-of-service (POS) health plans were distinct types of organizations and were identified as such. The term *managed*

Source: Adapted from E.R. Wagner, Types of Managed Care Organizations, in *The Managed Health Care Handbook,* 4th ed., P.R. Kongstvedt, ed., pp. 28–41, © 2000, Aspen Publishers, Inc. and P.R. Kongstvedt, Managed Health Care, in *Health Care Administration: Planning, Implementing, and Managing, Organized Delivery Systems,* 3rd ed., L.F. Wolper, ed., pp. 522–544, © 1999, Aspen Publishers, Inc.

care organization was not even used. Often lumped together as "alternative delivery systems," MCOs in the past two decades were a relatively small part of the health care landscape.

Now, far from being alternative delivery systems, MCOs are the predominant vehicles for the provision and payment of health care benefits, at least for the private sector. Furthermore, clear distinctions between types of health plans have become progressively blurred, and organizational elements that had appeared previously in only one type of MCO have found their way into other types of MCOs. As a result, it is now unusual to find MCOs that are pure examples of a type, and those that do exist are frequently organizations that serve only small, well-defined market areas (i.e., niche organizations), though there are some notable exceptions, such as Kaiser Permanente. More often, a seemingly pure MCO will be a subsidiary of a larger health plan or insurance company that offers other types of MCOs to the same market.

It is instructive to examine the different forms of MCOs, even if the boundaries between those forms are not clear in the current market. Although most MCOs have elements of more than one MCO type, they still generally fall into one of the standard classifications. It is also possible to further distinguish between MCOs that are primarily payers (e.g., health insurance companies and HMOs) and MCOs that are primarily provider-centered organizations.

TYPES OF BEARING RISK FOR MEDICAL COSTS

Contrary to popular belief, an insurance company or MCO does not necessarily bear all the financial risks associated with the medical costs of its clients or members. How an insurance company or MCO is structured or operates may be independent of the issue of financial risk for medical costs. There are three broad types of risk bearing from the standpoint of who pays the cost for health insurance (see Figure 2–1 and Exhibit 2–1): (1) government programs, (2) insurance, and (3) self-funded programs. Government programs and self-funded programs are briefly described here and discussed further in Chapters 6 and 7. Insurance is also briefly described here and is discussed throughout the entire book.

Government Programs

In the United States, the federal and state governments actually provide or finance more than 40 percent of health care. Government programs include Medicare for the elderly and disabled, Medicaid for the poor, military programs (both direct care by military providers and the TRICARE Program under the Civilian

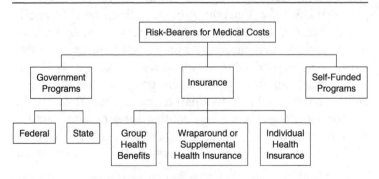

Figure 2–1 Risk-bearers for medical costs.

Exhibit 2–1 Risk-bearers for medical costs

---

1. Government Programs
   - Government (federal and/or state) bears risk for medical expenses unless it has contracted risk out to private health plans. Ultimately government agencies and taxpayers bear the risk.
   - Examples: Medicaid, Medicare, Federal Employees Health Benefit Program.
2. Insurance
   - Insurance company bears risk for medical expenses.
   - State governments set regulations regarding premiums charged to consumers or employers, benefits covered under policy, and privacy of health information.
   - Examples: Group health benefits plans, wraparound or supplemental health insurance, and individual health insurance.
3. Self-Funded Health Benefits Plans
   - Employers bear risk for medical expenses.
   - No state regulation. Employer must comply with federal requirements under ERISA.

Health and Medical Program of the Uniformed Services [CHAMPUS]), the Veterans Administration, the U.S. Public Health Service, and the Indian Health Service, among others. Some programs may incorporate only a few managed care features; others, several features; still others, all features.

The most important government programs are those that entitle certain eligible individuals to receive benefits from the government. These are called entitlement programs, and the primary examples are Medicare and Medicaid. The Centers for Medicare & Medicaid Services* (CMS), a branch of the

---

*As of July 1, 2001, the Health Care Financing Administration (HCFA) is now the Centers for Medicare & Medicaid Services (CMS) (http://www.cms.hhs.gov).

U.S. Department of Health and Human Services, administers Medicare, which provides health insurance for the elderly as well as for many individuals with end-stage renal disease. The states manage the Medicaid programs, which receive state and federal funds and provide health insurance to the poor and many disabled or institutionalized individuals.

Managed care techniques have been applied to all types of government programs, and there are, in fact, specific types of MCOs developed for Medicare and Medicaid. One special type of MCO for a government-sponsored program is the provider-sponsored organization (PSO), which is able to contract directly with CMS to provide prepaid medical services to a defined population of Medicare-eligible members who voluntarily enroll in the PSO. The PSO is a structurally unique type of MCO.

In all government entitlement programs, the risk for medical expenses is borne by state and/or federal government agencies and, ultimately, the taxpayers. This may be confusing to some individuals in the case of Medicare, because CMS contracts with private health plans, referred to as *intermediaries,* to administer the benefits of the Medicare program. In other words, the intermediary processes the claims of Medicare beneficiaries but does so only as an administrator, not as an insurance company at risk for medical expenses. To confuse things further, many private insurance companies offer Medicare beneficiaries so-called wraparound policies to pay for what Medicare does not cover; when the intermediary and the wraparound policy company are the same, it becomes difficult to understand who is responsible for what.

The Federal Employees Health Benefit Program (FEHBP) is a unique government program. Under this program, the federal government acts as an employer and makes health insurance plans or MCOs available to federal employees. Thus, the federal government is acting like any other employer in this regard. Consequently, the FEHBP is best understood, not as a government program, but as an employer-based group health benefits plan.

Insurance

People purchase health care insurance to protect themselves from unexpected medical costs. The insurer provides coverage of medical costs at a premium rate that is calculated to cover those costs on average. To differentiate health care insurance from government or self-funded health benefits plans, insurance is often referred to as "commercial" insurance (or "commercial" managed care in the case of an MCO).

The central point of health insurance is that the risk for medical expenses belongs to the insurance company. In other words, in exchange for the payment of insurance premiums, which can vary considerably in amount, the insurance company assumes the responsibility for paying the cost of medical benefits provided to individuals—that is, the cost of those benefits covered by the insurance policy in the first place. Other than the cost of the premium and any applicable co-payments (a fixed amount paid by the patient for each service) or coinsurance (a percentage of cost for service paid by insurance company with remaining percentage paid by patient) an insured individual is not at risk for the cost of medical care covered by the insurance policy.

With the notable exception of the Health Insurance Portability and Accountability Act (HIPAA; see Chapter 7), the federal government does not regulate the insurance industry. Rather, regulation of the industry is the responsibility of the state governments. The regulatory system is highly complex.

Each state taxes insurance via a premium tax; in other words, a small percentage of the premium charged to the purchaser is actually a tax. Most states have passed mandated benefits laws that require insurance policies to provide coverage for defined diseases, providers, procedures, and so forth. The states have different laws and regulations regarding privacy of health information and also regarding the manner in which insurance is actually sold (in order to ensure that each sale is fair and that the terms of coverage are fully disclosed).

They also have different laws and regulations regarding how and when certain types of premiums may be charged to particular types of consumers or employers. These are important issues because the medical expenses of everyone in the coverage "pool" affect the insurance premium rates. In other words, if one employer group has high medical costs, the premium rates for all of the other employer groups go up as well. The degree of that effect is determined by the type of policy.

Finally, it is common for insurance companies and MCOs, especially small to mid-sized health plans, to insure themselves against catastrophic costs. Thus, if the medical costs of the individuals and groups covered by the health plan become catastrophically high, the health plan has a reinsurance policy to cover some of the risk. This reinsurance policy "insures the insurer." Large insurance companies and MCOs usually do not need reinsurance policies because they have large financial reserves and can absorb changes in medical costs.

Group Health Benefits Plans

Employers generally purchase insurance policies to provide group health benefit plans for their eligible employees. Not all employees may be considered eligible, however; in fact, temporary or part-time employees are seldom eligible to participate in an employer's health insurance benefits plan. Group health benefits plans have several advantages:

- The cost of the insurance is paid on a pretax basis.
- Employers, especially large employers, are usually able to obtain more favorable pricing and coverage than individuals can.
- Health insurance benefits may be combined with other types of benefits (e.g., flexible spending accounts or life insurance).
- The employer, not the individual employee, manages administrative needs such as payroll deductions, payment of premiums, and so forth.

The most common type of group health benefits plan is the defined benefits insurance plan. In this type of plan, the benefits offered in the insurance policy are defined by what the employer has purchased on behalf of the employees. It is common for an employer to offer more than one type of defined benefits plan, however. For example, an employee may be able to choose (at different cost to the employee, of course) between a high-option insurance plan, a low-option insurance plan (i.e., with lesser levels of coverage), a managed care plan with more restrictions but higher benefits and lower costs, and so forth. The larger the employer is, the more likely that multiple health plans will be available to the employees.

If premium costs for a group health benefits plans increase, as they usually do each year, the employer generally absorbs all or some of that cost increase. The employees commonly must also contribute part of their pretax earnings toward the cost of the insurance. An employer may set that amount, referred to as a *payroll deduction,* to favor lower cost choices; for example, there may be no payroll deduction if the employee chooses an MCO, but the employee may have to pay the difference between the cost of the MCO and that of a more expensive insurance plan. In all cases, however, the payroll deduction is pretax, meaning that it is not considered income for purposes of calculating the employee's income tax.

An alternative to the defined benefits insurance plan is the defined contribution insurance plan. In this type of plan, the employer provides a fixed amount of money to the employees, who then purchase their own insurance, using both the defined contribution and their own money. This has the advantage to the employer of putting a lid on cost increases. The disadvantages are high for the employees, however, because the defined contribution may be considered ordinary taxable income, the cost of individual health insurance may be much higher than the cost of available group plans, and the contribution may be seen as inadequate. Variations of these two types of benefits plans—defined benefits and defined contribution—exist but are highly complex. The term *defined contribution* is often used to refer to a "fixed contribution" plan in which the employer selects a group of health benefits plan or plans, but fixes the amount the company will pay. Any increase in costs of the coverage must be paid by the employee.

Wraparound or Supplemental Health Insurance

An insurance policy that covers what another insurance policy does not cover is called a *wraparound* or *supplemental insurance policy*. For example, a group health benefits plan may have a $300 deductible and a lifetime limit on certain costs. It may even exclude coverage for certain conditions. A wraparound policy would provide the missing coverage (subject to its own limitations). The most common type of wraparound insurance policies are those that are sold to Medicare beneficiaries. Because Medicare has relatively high deductibles and coinsurance, the wraparound policy covers those costs. Also, Medicare does not provide coverage at all for certain expenses, such as costs of drugs or particular types of routine visits, and again the wraparound policy provides such coverage. Medicare wraparound policies must comply with requirements defined by CMS.

Individual Health Insurance

Individuals can purchase health insurance policies directly from commercial insurance companies. In general, individual health insurance policies are far more expensive and provide far less coverage than group policies. Exceptions are policies that are sold to young and healthy individuals, though changes in laws and regulations in many states have placed some limitations on how the premiums for young and healthy individuals may differ from those for older and sicker individuals. In many cases, unless they can meet certain strict criteria, individuals with existing medical problems may not even be able to buy health insurance.

Individuals who lose their jobs for any reason also lose their eligibility for the group health benefits plan offered by their former employer. Under the Consolidated Omnibus Reconciliation Act (COBRA), they are eligible to maintain their participation in the group policy at a small increase in cost over the group premium rate for up to 18 months, but only if they comply with strict requirements (e.g., for payment). Under HIPAA, they may also be eligible to purchase individual health insurance policies by meeting strict criteria, but the cost of such policies is usually quite high. Laws and regulations surrounding individual health insurance are highly complex and may differ from those surrounding group health benefits plans. Suffice it to say that individual health insurance is usually the least favorable option open to consumers, short of no insurance at all.

Self-Funded Health Benefits Plans

Many large corporations do not actually insure their employees at all in the sense that they do not purchase health insurance from an insurance company. They escape the burdens of purchasing insurance through self-funding as allowed by the Employee Retirement Income Security Act (ERISA). Assuming the risk of medical costs itself makes it possible for a large employer to avoid paying state premium tax and offering state mandated benefits; furthermore, the costs of its own group (its employees and their dependents) alone determine its costs. Self-funded benefits plans are not regulated by the states in any way, but they are regulated by the U.S. Department of Labor. As a practical matter, as long as an employer complies with the requirements under ERISA, there is very little regulation involved.

It is most common for a large employer to contract with a third-party administrator to perform the management activities required by the self-funded health benefits plan. Often, the third-party administrator is actually a large insurance company or a Blue Cross or Blue Shield plan, thus confusing in the minds of both members and providers who the insurer actually is. These large insurance companies provide not only administrative services but also substantial discounts to the employers when they receive such discounts from the providers. Self-funded plans may mimic any type of insurance coverage.

Almost every employer with a self-funded health benefits plan purchases reinsurance to protect itself from catastrophic medical costs. In other words, the self-funded plan actually does have some level of insurance, albeit very high-level insurance and only for extremely high costs. If the third-party administrator managing the self-funded health benefits plan is a large insurance company, a Blue Cross or Blue Shield plan, or an MCO, the third-party administrator itself may provide the reinsurance. If the third-party administrator is small or is not a large insurer in its own right, then the employer may purchase reinsurance directly. (As a complication, most states have rules regarding how much reinsurance a self-funded health benefits plan can have before it becomes commercial insurance and therefore subject to state regulation.)

PAYER-BASED MANAGED CARE

Managed care is an approach to managing both the quality and the cost of medical care. In the current environment, however, there really is no single definition of *managed care;* it is a term applied to a wide variety of systems. In general, managed care systems have at least two common elements: some type of authorization requirement and some level of restriction on a member's choice of providers. The authorization system may be minimal, requiring a simple hospital care precertification (i.e., advance approval), or it may be comprehensive, requiring a referral from a primary care physician (PCP) for any type of specialized care (i.e., "gatekeeper" model). The restriction on choice of provider may be minimal, such as a minor increase in coinsurance for seeing an out-of-network provider, or it may be severe, such as retraction of coverage for seeing an outside provider.

Managed care may be thought of as a continuum of models (Figure 2–2). These models are generally classified as follows:

- indemnity with precertification, mandatory second opinion, and case management
- service plan with precertification, mandatory second opinion, and case management
- preferred provider organization (PPO)
- point-of-service (POS) health plan
- "open-access" HMO
- traditional HMO
  1. open-panel HMO
     –independent practice association (IPA)
     –direct contract HMO

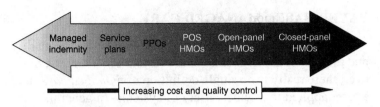

Figure 2–2 Continuum of managed care. Courtesy of William M. Mercer, Inc., San Francisco, California.

---

2. network model
3. closed-panel HMO
   –group model
   –staff model

As models move toward the managed care end of the continuum, the following features begin to appear:

- tighter elements of control over health care delivery
- addition of new elements of control
- more direct interaction with providers
- increased overhead cost and complexity
- greater control of utilization
- net reduction in rate of rise of medical costs

Although it would be comforting to classify all MCOs using the above models, the U.S. health care system has been mixing and matching the elements of these models to a dizzying degree. As noted earlier, MCOs are anything but uniform and rarely occur in a pure form.

The classification of health plans that follows has little to do with who carries the actual risk for medical expenses, which was the basis of the discussion of risk-bearing entities earlier in the chapter. The same terms may be used, but their meaning is different here. For instance, the terms *traditional insurance plan* and *service plan* now apply to certain kinds of health plans because of the structure and functioning of these plans, not their assumption of risk. To carry the example further, a traditional insurance plan may be either a truly traditional insurance plan in which the insurance company bears the risk for medical costs or a self-funded health benefits plan in which the employer bears the risk; from the viewpoint of a member or a provider, however, there is no difference.

Traditional Health Care Insurance

Basically, there are two types of traditional insurance: indemnity insurance and service plans. Note that although they are traditional, they have shrunk to occupy only a small fraction of the market for health care coverage.

Indemnity Insurance

Indemnity insurance protects the insured (i.e., the consumer or patient) against financial losses from medical expenses. The only restrictions are in the schedule of benefits listed in the insurance policy (i.e., what is covered by the policy). There are generally no restrictions on the licensed providers from whom the insured can seek care. The insurance company reimburses the subscriber directly for medical expenses or it may pay the provider directly, although it has no actual obligation other than to pay the subscriber. Payment to physicians and other professional providers is subject to usual, customary, or reasonable (UCR) fee screens, while payment to institutional providers is generally based on charges.

Benefits are generally subject to a deductible (a flat dollar amount that the subscriber must pay before the insurance company pays anything) and coinsurance (a percentage of the covered charge that the subscriber pays, such as 20 percent). Any charges by the provider that the insurance company does not pay are strictly the responsibility of the subscriber.

Most indemnity plans require precertification of elective hospital admissions and may apply a financial penalty to the subscriber who fails to obtain precertification. The plan may also require some additional utilization management of hospital cases, but plan-employed nurses working at another site generally take care of utilization issues over the telephone. Case management may also be used to help control the cost of catastrophic cases where costs are very high (severely premature infant or trauma cases). Second opinions may also be mandatory for certain elective procedures (e.g., cardiac bypass surgery).

The costs of this type of health care coverage have escalated faster than costs of any other type. As those costs have risen over the years, more people have moved into types of coverage that have a larger element of managed care.

Service Plans

The term *service plan* applies primarily, though not exclusively, to Blue Cross and Blue Shield Plans. In service plans, there are generally few restrictions on licensed providers who agree to sign a contract with the plan. The provider contract contains certain key provisions:

- The plan agrees to reimburse the provider directly, eliminating collection problems with patients.
- The provider agrees to accept the plan's fee schedule as payment in full and not to bill the subscriber for any payment not made by the plan (other than the normal deductible and coinsurance).
- The provider agrees to allow the plan to audit the provider's records.

Like indemnity insurance, service plans may require precertification, case management, and second opinions.

The principal advantage of a service plan over indemnity insurance is in the provider contracts and the reimbursement models that the contracts support. Professional fees allowed under the fee schedule may, in effect, provide a discount to the plan. More important, the plan usually has significant discounts at hospitals that give it a competitive advantage. The hospitals grant these discounts for a variety of reasons, including large volume of business, rapid payment, ease of collection, and, occasionally, advance deposits. The actual reimbursement to the hospital may be based on charges, diagnosis-related groups (DRGs), or some variation (see Chapter 3).

Preferred Provider Organizations

Although PPOs are similar to service plans, there are some important differences. A PPO may reduce the total panel of providers to some degree, often substantially (e.g., 30 percent of the total number of providers available in the area). There are two broad approaches that a PPO may take to establish a panel: "any willing provider" acceptance versus criteria-based selection. In the former, any provider who wishes to participate in the organization and who agrees to the terms and conditions of the PPO's contract must be offered a contract, at least until the PPO has adequate numbers of providers. In the latter, the PPO uses some objective criteria (e.g., credentials, practice pattern analysis) that a provider must meet before receiving a contract offer.

Although PPO payment mechanisms to providers may fall along the lines mentioned under service plans, the discounts are generally greater. Many service plans require providers to give them "most favored nation" pricing; in other words, a provider may not offer a better discount to a competitor than it does to the service plan. Such "favored nation" pricing has become less common recently because of regulatory and legal pressure.

Precertification, case management, and mandatory second opinion programs are almost always components of PPOs. The main difference between a PPO and a traditional health insurance plan is that failure to comply with these programs results in a financial penalty to the provider, not the subscriber. As with service plans, a contracting provider may not bill the subscriber for any balance that the PPO does not pay, except for the normal deductible and coinsurance. In the event that a subscriber chooses to seek care from a nonparticipating provider, the responsibility falls on the subscriber, and the subscriber is at risk for any charges not paid by the PPO.

A hallmark of a PPO is that benefits are reduced if a member seeks care from a provider who is not in the PPO network.

A common benefits differential is 20 percent. For example, if a member sees a network provider, coverage is provided at 90 percent of allowed charges; if a member sees a provider not in the network, the coverage may be at the 70-percent level.

PPOs can be either risk bearing or non-risk-bearing. A risk-bearing PPO combines the insurance, or payment, function with the management of the network of providers. A non-risk-bearing PPO focuses solely on network management, not on the insurance function. For example, a commercial insurer may build a network and sell coverage to clients; this insurer is a risk-bearing PPO. Alternatively, a group of providers may come together as a legal entity, establish professional principles (e.g., fee allowances, credentialing criteria, utilization review), and contract with independent insurers to provider medical services to those insurers' customers; this organization is a non-risk-bearing PPO.

Health Maintenance Organizations

HMOs are fundamentally different from the health plans described above. Although there are a few exceptions known as "open-access" HMOs that are similar in benefits design to PPOs, the vast majority of HMOs manage utilization and quality to a greater degree than PPOs. Benefits to members in an HMO are restricted (with some exceptions) to services executed by the HMO's providers in compliance with the HMO's authorization procedures. Benefits obtained through the HMO tend to be significantly more generous than those found in a traditional insurance plan or a PPO. Except in true emergencies or specifically authorized instances, payment for services received from non-HMO providers is the responsibility of the subscriber, not the HMO. Services executed by contracted providers who fail to obtain proper authorization are the responsibility of the provider, who may not bill the subscriber for any fees not paid by the HMO.

Traditional HMOs currently fall into two broad categories: open panel and closed panel. A third category, the true network model, is uncommon except in certain parts of the country, but may become more widespread in the future (Figure 2–3). Some HMOs combine or mix different model types in the same market. Since open-access HMOs are not considered traditional HMOs, they are discussed separately, followed by a discussion of traditional open- and closed-panel plans.

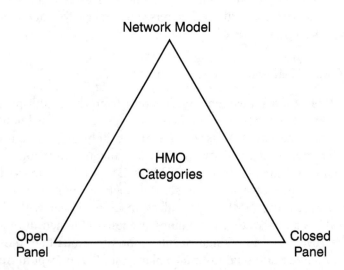

Figure 2–3 Types of HMOs.

Open-Access HMOs

Open access HMOs are more like PPOs than traditional HMOs. In the open-access HMO model, members may access any provider in the HMO without going through a primary care physician (PCP). Thus, members may see any PCP or specialist in the network on a self-referral basis. The physicians in the open-access HMO share at least some level of risk for costs. Therefore, if professional costs exceed the budget, the physicians accept lower fees, lose their withholds (i.e., the amount of payment that the HMO holds back to cover higher than budgeted medical costs) and so forth. In this model, it is theoretically possible to pay specialists a capitation fee (i.e., a set fee paid each month for each member), but it is extremely hard in practice because there is no reliable base to use for the capitation (i.e., members are not required to select specific PCPs or specialists, so the actuaries cannot decide who should receive the capitation payment).

Open-access plans were popular in the late 1970s and early 1980s, especially plans sponsored by organized medical societies. With a few exceptions, these plans suffered substantial losses and failed. There has been a recent revival of interest in open-access plans, however, because of consumer demands. Such demands are certainly logical: who does not want a health care plan with a high level of benefits, low costs, and unlimited access to providers? The HMOs that are currently adopting open-access designs are doing so on the assumption that, because so few referral authorizations are denied, the referral requirement is not worth the cost. This line of reasoning ignores the value of asking a PCP to judge whether a referral is necessary rather than relying on a patient to make that judgment; in other words, it is assumed either that most patient requests for referrals will be appropriate or that PCPs will generally not refuse to grant the requests. Although open-access HMOs failed miserably in past years, it remains unknown if they will fare better now that physicians and hospitals are functioning more efficiently than in the past.

Open-Panel Plans

In an open-panel HMO, private physicians and other professional providers are independent contractors who see HMO members in their own offices. They may contract with more than one competing health plan (and usually do) and also see fee-for-service patients. A variety of reimbursement mechanisms may be used. The total number of providers in an open-panel plan is larger than that in a closed-panel plan but usually smaller than in a PPO. Each member must choose a single provider to be his or her PCP (sometimes referred to as a "gatekeeper"), who must authorize any other services. Members may change their PCPs at designated times if they wish.

Open-panel plans fall into two broad categories: independent practice associations (IPAs) and direct contract models. Although the terms are often used synonymously, the two models are technically distinct. In an IPA model, the HMO contracts with a legal entity known as an IPA and pays it a negotiated capitation amount. The IPA, in turn, contracts with private physicians to provide health care to the HMO members. The IPA may pay the physicians through capitation or may use another mechanism, such as fee-for-service. The providers are at risk under this model in that if medical costs exceed the capitation amount, the IPA receives no additional funds from the HMO and must accordingly adjust its payments to the providers.

In the direct contract model, the HMO contracts directly with the providers; there is no intervening entity. The HMO pays the providers directly and performs all related management tasks. Direct contract HMOs are currently the most common type.

Closed-Panel Plans

Unlike physicians in an open-panel plan, physicians in a closed-panel plan confine their practice to the HMO members. These physicians practice in facilities that are likewise dedicated to the HMO. The total number of providers in the closed-panel plan is by far the smallest of any model type. Members usually do not have to choose a single PCP but may see any PCP or any physician in the HMO facility; however, they may be asked to choose a primary facility in order to ensure continuity of care.

Closed-panel plans fall into two broad categories: group model and staff model. In a group model plan, the HMO contracts with a group of physicians to provide services to members. The HMO pays the group a negotiated capitation amount, and the group in turn pays the individual physicians through a combination of salary and risk/reward incentives. The group is responsible for its own governance, and the physicians are either partners in the group or associates. The group or the HMO may provide the dedicated practice facilities and support staff, but most commonly the HMO assumes that responsibility. The group is at risk in that, if the costs of the group exceed the capitation amount, the reimbursement to the providers is less—although the HMO generally provides stop-loss reinsurance to the group to protect the group from catastrophic cost overruns. Some groups exist primarily on paper and actually operate strictly as cost pass-through (i.e., the costs are simply passed from the medical group to the HMO, and the group does not actually bear any risk for medical expenses) vehicles for the HMO; in this event, the arrangement resembles a staff model plan.

In a staff model plan, the HMO contracts with the providers directly, and the providers are employees of the HMO. Physicians receive a salary, and there is an incentive plan of some sort. The HMO has full responsibility for the management of all activities.

Network Model HMOs

Occasionally, the term *network model* is used to refer to an open-panel plan, but in the "true" network model, the HMO contracts with several large multispecialty medical groups for services. The groups receive payment under capitation, and they in turn pay the physicians under a variety of mechanisms. The groups operate relatively independently. The HMO contracts with more than one group, but the number of groups is usually limited.

Mixed Model HMOs

Nothing in this world is pure and simple, and health plans are no exception. Many HMOs have adopted several model types, even in the same market, in order to attract as many members as possible and capture additional market share. The most common form of mixed model involves grafting a direct contract model onto either a closed-panel or a network model.

For example, the HMO may need to expand its medical service area and may choose to contract with private physicians rather than make the expenditures required for an additional facility. In mixed model plans, the models often operate independently of each other.

Point-of-Service Plans

Plans based on the point of service (POS) combine features of HMOs and traditional insurance plans. In a POS plan, members may choose which system to use at the point they obtain the service. For example, if a member uses his or her PCP and otherwise complies with the HMO authorization system, the benefits for services may be quite generous, and the member would be required to pay only a minor copayment. If the member chooses to self-refer or otherwise not to use the HMO system to receive services, the plan still provides insurance coverage but would require a higher deductible and higher coinsurance. The difference between coverage for in-network services and out-of-network services generally ranges from 20 percent to 40 percent.

Point-of-service plans have developed because of the conflict between cost control and total freedom of choice of providers. By bringing the issue of cost differential directly to HMO members at the point where they seek medical services, the members become a more active participants in the process.

INTEGRATED DELIVERY SYSTEMS

Like MCOs, organized health care delivery systems, also know as *integrated delivery systems* (IDSs), fall into various categories. (Some legal and tax professionals prefer to reserve the term *integrated delivery system* for distinct corporate entities that operate under a single identity for purposes of taxation and liability. This book makes no such distinction.) Most IDSs have been established to make it easier for different types of providers to work together in a managed care environment. IDSs contract with MCOs, coordinate the care delivered to patients, and enhance efficiencies in the health care delivery system overall. The success of IDSs in meeting these goals has been mixed at best, and many large IDSs have failed in the recent past. Other IDSs have achieved some of the goals, however, in particular the goals that are generally easier to achieve by larger organizations with correspondingly greater negotiating leverage.

Like the classification system for MCOs, the classification system for IDSs is imprecise. Furthermore, the terms used to describe IDSs rival those in the rest of the managed care industry for sheer number and vagueness of definition. Following is a list of names and acronyms for some of the main types of IDSs:

- independent practice association (IPA)
- physician-hospital organization (PHO)
- management services organization (MSO)
- provider-sponsored organization (PSO)
- physician practice management company (PPMC)
- group practice without walls (GPWW)
- medical group practice
- foundation model
- staff model

- virtual integration
- other weird arrangement (OWA)

Multiple IDSs may exist within any single health care delivery system, and the definition and actual activities of an IDS may not be the same from one organization to another. For example, an IDS may contain an IPA to organize independent physicians, a PPMC to manage the physician practices owned by the hospital, a PHO to serve as the contracting vehicle for the IDS's contracts with MCOs, and so forth. The following is a brief description of the most common types of IDSs or components of IDSs.

Independent Practice Association

IPAs have been in existence for several decades The members of an IPA are independent physicians who contract with the IPA, which is a legal entity, so that the IPA can contract with one or more HMOs. Although most IPAs are nonprofit, some are for-profit. The term *independent practice association* is often used to refer to any type of open-panel HMO, but this usage is not technically correct.

In a typical case, the IPA negotiates with an HMO for a capitation rate that takes into account all physician services. The IPA, in turn, pays the member physicians, although not necessarily according to a capitation rate. The IPA and its member physicians are at risk for at least some portion of medical costs in that, if the capitation rate is too low to cover the physician payments, the physicians must accept a lower income. It is the presence of this risk sharing that distinguishes the IPA from a negotiating vehicle that does not bear risk. It is also the reason that a true IPA is not typically subject to anti-trust lawsuits (unless it was formed solely or primarily to keep out competition). Usually, an IPA is an umbrella organization for physicians in all specialties to participate in managed care. Recently, however, IPAs representing only a single specialty have emerged.

An IPA may operate simply as a negotiating organization, with the HMO providing all administrative support, or it may take on some of the duties of the HMO, such as utilization management or network development. In some cases, particularly if the IPA is large and mature, the IPA may also adjudicate claims. The IPA generally has stop-loss reinsurance (or is provided such insurance by the HMO) to avoid going bankrupt (see Chapter 3).

Physician-Hospital Organization

By definition, a PHO requires the participation of a hospital and at least some portion of the admitting physicians. Often, the hospital proposes the formation of the PHO, but unless the leadership of the medical staff supports it, the idea is unlikely to get far. It is not uncommon for a PHO to be formed primarily as a mechanism for dealing with an increase in managed care contracting activity. It is also not uncommon for the same physicians who join the PHO already to be under contract with one or more managed care plans.

At a minimum, the PHO is an entity that allows a hospital and its affiliated physicians to negotiate with MCOs. In its weakest form, it operates as a "messenger." The PHO analyzes the terms and conditions offered by an MCO and transmits the analysis and the contract to each physician, who then decides on an individual basis whether to participate.

Typically, the participating physicians and the hospital develop model contract terms and reimbursement levels and use those to negotiate with MCOs. The PHO usually has a limited amount of time to negotiate a contract successfully (e.g., 90 days). If the time limit passes without an agreement, then the participating physicians are free to contract directly with the MCO. If the PHO successfully reaches an agreement with the MCO, then the physicians agree to be bound by the terms of the PHO's contract with the MCO. Confusingly, the actual contract for health care services is still between the physician and the MCO or between the hospital and the MCO. In some cases, the contract between the physicians and the MCO is relatively concise and may refer to the contract between the PHO and the MCO.

The PHO may actively manage the relationship between the providers and MCOs. It is usually a separate business entity, such as a for-profit corporation. Issues such as how equity or ownership is divided between the physicians and the hospital, where the money comes from to operate the PHO, how (or even if) money comes into the PHO from its managed care activities—these are all complex issues that must be resolved.

One last note regarding PHOs: The physician portion may itself be a different type of IDS, such as a GPWW or an IPA. Although currently the most common model is one in which the physicians remain independent and contract individually with the PHO, the use of IPAs has been increasing. There are other methods of organization as well.

Management Services Organization

The MSO represents the evolution of the PHO into an entity that provides more management services to the physicians. Not only does the MSO provide a vehicle for negotiating with MCOs, but also it also offers additional services to support the physicians' practices. The physicians, however, usually remain independent private practitioners. An MSO is based around one or more hospitals. The reasons for an MSO's formation are generally the same as those for the formation of a PHO (primarily contract negotiation), and the ownership and operational issues are similar.

In its simplest form, an MSO operates as a service bureau, providing basic practice support services to member physicians. These services include billing and collection, administrative support in certain areas, and electronic data interchange. The physicians can remain independent practitioners, under no legal obligation to use the services of the hospital on an exclusive basis. The MSO must receive payment from the physicians at fair market value for the services that the MSO does provide, however, or the hospital and the physicians could incur legal problems.

Some MSOs may be considerably broader in scope. In addition to providing all the services that have been described, an MSO may actually purchase many of the assets of a physician's practice. For example, the MSO may purchase the physician's office space or office equipment (at fair market value), can employ the office support staff of the physician, and can even perform functions such as quality management, utilization management, provider relations, member services, and claims processing. An MSO of this type is usually constructed as a unique business entity separate from a PHO.

A MSO does not always directly contract with MCOs, for two reasons. First, many MCOs insist that the providers themselves be the contracting agents (to be sure that the providers understand and agree to the contractual terms, and to make sure that the contract remains in force even if the MSO ceases to exist). Second, many states will not allow MCOs (especially HMOs) to have contracts with any entity that does not have the power to bind the provider, something an MSO may not be able to do because the physicians may remain independent private practitioners (i.e., as independent providers, they could refuse to honor the contract terms unless they sign it themselves.). There are IDSs calling themselves management services organizations that actually do purchase entire physician practices (possibly including intangible values such as good will) and function much like a fully integrated system.

Provider-Sponsored Organization

Generally, a PSO is a cooperative venture of a group of providers who control the venture's health service delivery and financial arrangements. In effect, a PSO is an integrated provider system engaged in both delivering and financing health care services. Its focus is typically on the Medicare population, but it could theoretically expand to include commercial and Medicaid initiatives as well.

The Balanced Budget Act of 1997 created PSOs through a set of provisions referred to as Medicare+Choice (see Chapter 6). The Medicare+Choice provisions of the Balanced Budget Act contain the following definition:

A PSO is a public or private entity that is a provider or group of affiliated providers that provides a substantial portion of health care under the contract directly through the provider or affiliated group of providers, and with respect to those affiliated providers that share, directly or indirectly, substantial financial risk, have at least a majority interest in the entity.

In an urban area, a substantial portion of health care services is defined as 70 percent or more (as measured by expenditures); in a rural area, it is defined as 60 percent or more.

When the act created PSOs, there was a general belief that they would eliminate the administrative overhead costs associated with Medicare HMOs and that providers themselves would be better positioned to manage both the cost and the quality of health care for Medicare beneficiaries. These assumptions proved to be false, however, and the few PSOs that came into existence failed within a few years, experiencing spectacular losses and creating substantial managerial pain within the provider systems themselves.

Physician Practice Management Company

In the mid-1990s, PPMCs arrived on the scene, and they acquired physician practices throughout the middle to late 1990s. PPMCs may be viewed as variant MSOs, but unlike the MSOs described earlier, PPMCs are for physicians only. In other words, hospitals have no involvement. Some authorities refer to these organizations as physician-only MSOs.

In general, a PPMC manages all support functions (e.g., billing and collections, purchasing, contract negotiations) but remains relatively uninvolved with the clinical aspects of a physician's practice. In many cases, the physician remains an independent practitioner, although the PPMC owns all the tangible assets of the practice. The PPMC usually takes a percentage of the practice revenue, often at a rate equal to or slightly below the physician's previous overhead costs. The physician makes a long-term commitment to the PPMC and agrees not to compete with the other physicians if he or she leaves the company.

It was hoped that PPMCs, usually organized on a for-profit basis, would achieve more efficient management and economies of scale, thereby producing a profit while maintaining physician income. Practice acquisitions were expected to give PPMCs a stronger negotiating position vis-à-vis MCOs, at least when a PPMC represented a substantial percentage of the physicians in a given area. Many PPMCs also sought global capitation contracts (i.e., contracts covering administrative and medical services), and in general they desired to cut out the hospital from any profit and control.

Some practitioners, exasperated by the pressures of running a practice, preferred selling their practices to a PPMC rather than a hospital, possibly because they distrusted the hospital or expected the PPMC to have greater practice management capability. Unfortunately, in most cases, these physicians have been disappointed. Not only did the PPMCs fail to demonstrate the management expertise that the physicians expected, but the practice acquisitions made the physicians employees (or employee-like staff members) for many years, with all the attendant motivational effects.

In general, the track record of PPMCs is terrible, and they fell to ruin in large numbers. Most major PPMCs have disappeared, either through bankruptcy or by exiting the business. Because some PPMCs are doing well, it is not appropriate to dismiss the concept out of hand. Like the PSOs, the PPMC may yet be resurrected, but currently it is not a significant type of IDS.

Group Practice Without Walls

Also known as the clinic without walls, the GPWW is a step toward greater integration of small physician practices. It does not require the participation of a hospital and indeed is often the result of physicians' desire to organize without being dependent on a hospital for services or support. In some cases, GPWW formation has occurred to take advantage of the strength that numbers give in negotiating with MCOs and with hospitals.

A GPWW is composed of private practice physicians who agree to combine their practices into a single legal entity but continue to practice medicine in their independent locations. In other words, the physicians appear to be independent from the point of view of their patients, but they are a single group from the point of view of a contracting entity (usually an MCO). Two features differentiate GPWWs from PPMCs: first, the GPWW is owned solely by the member physicians and not by any outside investors, and second, the GPWW is a legal merging of all assets of the physician practices rather than the acquisition of only the tangible assets (as is often the case in an PPMC).

The member physicians own and govern the GPWW. They may contract with an outside organization for business support services. Office support services are generally provided through the group, although the physicians may notice little difference in their day-to-day office procedures.

For various legal and organizational reasons, the GPWW is a model that has not become common, much less dominant. Many state and federal enforcement agencies have concluded that without significant sharing of operations and financial risk, that GPWWs exist solely for anti-competitive price negotiating, causing the GPWW to either become a real group practice, or to dissolve

Medical Group Practice

Traditionally, physicians who have wanted to combined their resources have done so in truly unified medical group practices. Unlike the GPWW, in which the physicians combine certain assets and risks but continue to practice medicine in their own offices, the true medical group has one or a small number of locations and functions as a group. That is, there is a great deal of interaction among the members of the group, as well as common goals and objectives.

Traditional medical groups are legally independent of hospitals. Even so, it is common for a group to identify strongly with one hospital. Although this is good for the hospital as long as relations are good, it can be devastating if relations sour or if the group decides to change hospitals for any reason. Some hospitals sponsor medical groups, but those groups operate more like staff models.

A medical group is usually a partnership or professional corporation, although other forms are possible. Usually, the more senior members of the group enjoy more of the fruits of the group's success (e.g., higher income, better on-call schedules). An existing group often requires new members to pass a probationary period and to make a substantial contribution to the group's capital upon joining, which can create an entry barrier and retard growth. Other groups simply employ new physicians for a lengthy period in order to control the finances of the group (new physicians are paid considerably less than senior physicians) as well as give all parties the opportunity to see whether they can work together successfully. In any event, it is common for a medical group to require a noncompete clause in each physician's contract to protect the group from physician defections and the taking away of patients.

In a medical group, the performance of the group as a whole affects the personal income of the member physicians. Although an IPA places a defined portion of a physician's income at risk (that portion related to the managed care contract held by the IPA), the medical group's income from any source determines the individual physician's income and profit; that being said, an individual physician's productivity is commonly the most important factor in determining his or her income while part of a medical group.

Foundation Model

In one type of foundation model IDS, a hospital creates a nonprofit foundation and actually purchases physician practices (both tangible and intangible assets) and puts those practices into the foundation. This model usually occurs when the hospital cannot employ the physicians directly or use hospital funds to purchase the practices directly (as might be the case if the hospital is a nonprofit entity that cannot own a for-profit subsidiary or if a state law prohibits the corporate practice of medicine). To qualify for and maintain its nonprofit status, the foundation must prove that it provides substantial benefits to the community.

A second form of foundation model does not involve a hospital. In that model, the foundation is an independent entity that contracts for services with a medical group and a hospital. On a historical note, in the early days of HMOs, many open-panel plans that were not formed as IPAs were formed as foundations; the foundation held the HMO license and contracted with one or more IPAs and hospitals for services.

The foundation itself is governed by a board that is not dominated by either the hospital or the physicians (in fact, physician representation on the board is not allowed to be above 20 percent). The board includes lay members. The foundation owns and manages the practices, but the physicians become members of a medical group that in turn has an exclusive contract for services with the foundation; in other words, the foundation is the only source of revenue for the medical group. The physicians have long-term contracts with the medical group, and the contracts contain noncompete clauses.

Although the physicians are in an independent group and the foundation is independent from the hospital, the relationship between the three is close. The medical group, however, retains a significant measure of autonomy regarding its own business affairs, and the foundation has no control over certain aspects, such as individual physician compensation.

Staff Model

The distinction between the staff model associated with an HMO, as discussed earlier, and that associated with an IDS owned by a health system is whether the principal business organization is a risk-bearing, licensed entity (e.g., an HMO) or primarily a provider. The staff model is a health system that employs the physicians directly. Physicians enter the system either through the purchase of their practices or through direct recruitment. The system usually comprises more than just a hospital; it is a large, comprehensive health care organization. Because the physicians are employees, the legal issues attached to IDSs using private physicians are reduced.

Virtual Integration

Goldsmith* has argued that many of the structurally rigid vertical integration models are not going to succeed. In his opinion, success will be more likely with models of virtual integration, in which more or less independent parties come together and behave like an IDS under managed care but retain their own identities and mission. This virtual integration requires an alignment of the financial incentives among the parties as well as an alignment of their business goals.

In virtual integration, each of the major segments of the health care system—the physicians, the institutional providers, the payers (or MCOs), and the ancillary providers (e.g.,

---

*J.C. Goldsmith, The Illusive Logic of Integration, *Healthcare Forum Journal,* September-October 1994, 26–31.

pharmacies)—act in concert for a common cause, but none is an employee or subdivision of another. Each party manages its own affairs and meets its own financial goals without being managed by another segment of the industry. In this model, there is greater horizontal integration (e.g., between hospitals, between physicians), and each of the horizontally integrated groups then forms relationships with other parts of the health care system.

Other Weird Arrangement

Any type of organization that defies easy description qualifies as an other weird arrangement (OWA)—the catchall category for innovative approaches. The lifespan of most OWAs tends to be very short.

GOVERNANCE AND MANAGEMENT OF MCOS

The governance and management of an MCO is influenced by its type, its structure (or that of its parent company), and many other variables. The function of key officers or managers as well as of committees depends on the MCO's type, its ownership, and the motivations and skills of the individuals involved. Further, MCOs must comply with many legal and regulatory requirements (state and federal), and which requirements apply depends on the MCO's structure and features (e.g., whether it is for-profit or nonprofit; whether it is provider owned; its state of domicile; and what types of products it offers). Thus, each health care system must construct its own management control structure to suit its own needs.

Board of Directors

Many but not all managed care plans have a board of directors. Numerous factors influence the composition and function of the board, which has the final responsibility for the plan's operation. Plans that do not necessarily have their own boards include the following:

- PPOs developed by large insurance companies
- PPOs developed for single employers by an insurance company
- HMOs set up by a single company just for the purpose of serving the company's employees
- Employer-sponsored or -developed plans (PPOs, precertification operations)
- HMOs or exclusive provider organizations set up by an insurance company as a line of business

With one exception, each of these entities is a subsidiary of a larger company, and whereas the company does have a board of directors, the board oversees the entire company, not just the subsidiary. A PPO or HMO that is a division of an insurance company may be required to list a board on its licensure forms, but that board may have little real operational role. The one exception, as noted earlier, is an HMO set up by a single company to serve its employees; such an HMO is considered to be self-funded and is regulated by labor laws, not insurance laws.

Although most HMOs have boards of directors, not all of those boards are completely functional. This is especially true for HMOs that are part of large national companies. Each local HMO is incorporated and required by law to have a board, but it is not uncommon for the national company to use the same corporate officers as the board for every local HMO. Though the board fulfills its legal function and obligation, control of the actual operation of the HMO comes through the management structure of the national company rather than through a direct relationship between the HMO executives and the board.

Membership

The composition of the board of directors varies depending on whether the plan is for-profit (in which case the owners' or shareholders' representatives may hold the majority of seats) or nonprofit (in which case community representation will be broader). Some nonprofit health plans are organized as cooperatives (i.e., a legal entity in which the members, or enrollees, are as a group in control of the entity), in which case the board members are all members of the plan. In nonprofit plans that are not cooperatives, board members generally should be truly independent and have no potential conflicts of interest; provider-sponsored nonprofit plans may restrict seats held by providers to no more than 20 percent. In any case, local events, company bylaws, and laws and regulations (including the tax code for nonprofit health plans) dictate whether the board members come from outside the health plan or from the staff of the plan. Because in a provider-sponsored for-profit plan the providers may have majority representation, they must take special precautions to avoid antitrust problems; for example, an objective outside party rather than the providers themselves must set fees.

Responsibilities

The function of an MCO board of directors is governance—overseeing the MCO's activities. Final approval of corporate bylaws rests with the board. It is the bylaws that determine the basic structure of power, both that of the plan officers and that of the board itself. Because significant liability issues surround the board of directors, each board member must undertake his or her duties with care and diligence.

The fiduciary responsibility of the board of directors (i.e., their duty to protect the organization's financial assets) is clear. The board's duties include not only general oversight of the MCO's profitability or reserve status (money in reserve for when costs exceed premium income) but also approval of significant fiscal events, such as a major acquisition or expenditure. In a for-profit plan, the board has fiduciary responsibility to protect the interests of the stockholders.

As part of their legal responsibilities, members of the board may have to review certain reports and sign particular documents. For example, a board officer may be required to sign the quarterly financial report to the state regulatory agency, and the board chairperson may be required to sign any acquisition documents. The board is also responsible for the veracity of financial statements sent to stockholders.

Policy making is another common function of an active board. This responsibility may be as broad as determining whether to use a gatekeeper system, or it may be as detailed as approving organization charts and reporting structures. Although the plan officers set most of the day-to-day policies and procedures, an active board may set a policy regarding what operational policies the officers must bring to the board for approval or change.

In HMOs and many other types of MCOs, the board of directors has special responsibilities in several areas. First is the oversight of the quality of care delivered to members and the quality management program. Usually, the board carries out this responsibility through a review of the quality management documentation (including the overall quality management plan and regular reports on findings and activities), either by the full board or a board subcommittee, and through feedback to the medical director and plan quality management committee. Second is corporate compliance with privacy requirements under HIPAA and with Medicare requirements for those MCOs with Medicare contracts.

In free-standing plans, the board also has responsibility for hiring the chief executive officer (CEO) of the plan and for reviewing that officer's performance. The board in such plans often sets the CEO's compensation package, and the CEO reports to the board.

Active boards generally have committees for certain functions, including an executive committee (e.g., to make decisions rapidly), a compensation committee (e.g., to set general compensation guidelines for the plan's staff, set the CEO's compensation, and approve and issue stock options), a finance committee or audit committee (e.g., to review financial statistics, approve budgets, set and approve spending authority, review the annual audit, review and approve outside funding sources), a corporate compliance committee, and a quality management committee.

Key Management Positions

The roles and titles of the key managers in any organization vary depending on the type of organization, its legal status, its line of business, its complexity, and whether it is a free-standing entity or a satellite of another operation, among other factors. There is little consistency from health plan to health plan. How each key role is defined (or even whether it is present at all) is strictly up to the management of each plan. Thus, it is possible to provide only a general overview of certain key roles (Figure 2–4).

Executive Director

Most plans have at least one key manager. Sometimes called an executive director, a CEO, a general manager, or a plan manager, this individual is usually responsible for all the

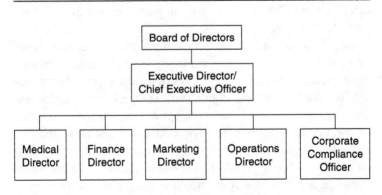

Figure 2–4 Key management positions in a health plan.

operational aspects of the plan. This is not always the case, however. For example, some large companies (e.g., insurance companies or national HMO chains) have their local marketing directors report directly to a regional marketing director rather than to the local plan manager. A few companies take that to the extreme of having the chief of every functional area report to regional managers instead of to a single local manager. Thus, reporting is a function of the overall environment, and there is little standardization in the industry.

In free-standing plans and traditional HMOs, the executive director is responsible for all areas. The other officers and key managers report to the executive director, who in turn reports to the board (or to a regional manager in the case of national companies). The executive director also has responsibility for general administrative operations and public relations.

Medical Director

It can almost be assumed that managed care plans will have a medical director. The needs of the plan determine whether that position is full-time or filled by a community physician who comes in a few hours a week. The medical director usually has responsibility for provider relations, provider recruiting, quality management, utilization management, and medical policy.

In some plans (e.g., simple PPOs), the medical director alone, or a medical consultant, may review claims, approve physician applications, and examine patterns of utilization. The intensity of medical director involvement parallels the level of medical management. Usually, the medical director reports to the executive director.

Finance Director

In free-standing plans or large operations, it is common to have a finance director or chief financial officer. That individual is generally responsible for all financial and accounting operations. In some plans, these operations include functions such as billing, management information services (MIS), enrollment, and underwriting (analyzing groups to determine rates and benefits) as well as accounting, fiscal reporting, and budget preparation. The person in this position usually reports to the executive director, although once again some national companies require reporting to a higher level.

Marketing Director

The responsibility for marketing the plan belongs to the marketing director. Responsibility generally includes oversight of marketing representatives, advertising, client relations, and enrollment forecasting. A few plans have the marketing department generate initial premium rates, which are then sent to the finance or underwriting department for review, but that is uncommon. The marketing director reports to the executive director or to someone at a higher level, depending on the company.

Operations Director

In larger plans, it is not uncommon to have an operations director. The person in this position usually oversees claims, MIS, enrollment, underwriting (unless finance is doing so), member services, office management, and any other traditional back room functions. The operations director usually reports to the executive director.

Corporate Compliance Officer

As mentioned previously, health plans have certain corporate compliance requirements. HIPAA contains extensive privacy requirements that an MCO must meet, and the MCO must appoint a specific individual responsible for ensuring the organization is in compliance with these requirements. Similarly, an MCO with a Medicare+Choice risk contract needs a corporate compliance officer to ensure compliance with Medicare requirements. One corporate compliance officer may be able to fulfill all of these responsibilities.

Committees

Again, there is little consistency from organization to organization regarding committees. Most organizations have nonmedical standing committees to address management issues in defined areas. In contrast, ad hoc committees, by definition, are convened to meet a specific need and then dissolved. A consumer or member advisory committee is common type of nonmedical committee; although its members have no voting rights or governance powers, they provide consumer or member input to plan managers. In the medical management area, committees serve to diffuse some elements of responsibility (which can be beneficial for medical-legal reasons) and allow important input from providers into procedures and policies or even into case-specific interpretations of existing policies.

Quality Management Committee

Usually required under law and/or for accreditation purposes, the quality management committee is essential for overseeing quality management, standard setting, data review, feedback to providers, follow-up, and approval of sanctions. A peer review committee may be a subcommittee of the quality management committee or it may be separate.

Credentialing Committee

Health plans generally have a credentialing committee charged with ensuring that the providers have the necessary professional qualifications (i.e., credentials) to participate in the plan. This committee may be a subcommittee of the quality management committee or it may be separate. In new plans with extensive credentialing needs, it is probably best for the committee to be separate. In states that have carefully defined "due process" requirements for provider termination, this is the committee most likely to take on the responsibility for compliance with those requirements.

Medical Advisory Committee

The purpose of a medical advisory committee is to review general medical management issues brought to it by the medical director. Such issues may include changes in the contract with providers, in compensation, or in authorization procedures. This committee serves as a sounding board for the medical director. Occasionally, it has decision-making authority, but that is rare because such authority really belongs to the board of directors. In national companies, a local committee may have input for local medical management issues, but a corporate-level medical policy committee generally resolves medical issues that cross all plans (e.g., medical policies regarding new technology).

Utilization Review Committee

The medical director may bring utilization issues to the utilization review committee. Often this committee is responsible for policies regarding plan coverage. This committee is also the one that reviews the utilization patterns of the providers and may impose sanctions on providers who use medical resources inappropriately or unwisely.

Sometimes, in reviewing cases for medical necessity, the utilization review committee helps to resolve disputes between the plan and a provider regarding utilization. In large plans, this function may be placed in the hands of various specialty panels charged with reviewing the utilization of consultants (i.e., specialty physicians). The committee may be part of the medical advisory committee or it may be free-standing.

Pharmacy and Therapeutics Committee

Plans that offer significant pharmacy benefits to their members often have a pharmacy and therapeutics committee. This committee is usually charged with developing a formulary (a list of drugs approved for prescription by plan physicians), reviewing changes to the formulary, and examining abnormal prescription utilization patterns by providers. This committee is usually free-standing. In national MCOs, the formulary may or may not be subject to local input, depending on the plan benefits (e.g., whether plan members have different copayments for generic drugs versus brand-name drugs).

Medical Grievance Review Committee

In most states and for members covered under any federal health plan, including Medicare, health care plans must establish a separate committee to review member grievances that pertain to medical management or coverage determinations. A particular grievance must be investigated mostly by health care professionals whose specialty encompasses the medical condition at issue, and therefore most health care professional members will attend a committee meeting only if their specialty is appropriate to the grievance under review. The health care professionals investigating the grievance should not have participated in the member's medical care; if the grievance is significant, it may be necessary to have practitioners who are not associated with the plan look at the validity of the grievance.

Related to the grievance review process is the process for external review of appeals. In states that do not require external reviews, the reviews may be performed by a contracted group of independent physicians. In states that do, the states themselves usually define the independent review organization and require that it not be part of the plan's committee structure. As yet, the federal government does not require the external review of appeals, but this may change.

Corporate Compliance Committee

Corporate compliance activities are directed toward ensuring conformance to legal and regulatory requirements and preventing and detecting illegal behavior. Corporate compliance programs usually include a special compliance committee that is responsible for creating standards of conduct for employees and also creating policies and procedures specifically designed to ensure compliance with pertinent regulations, such as the Medicare+Choice rules. Further discussion of corporate compliance is found in Chapter 6.

CONCLUSION

An understanding of the common types of MCOs and IDSs, as well as their basic management, is required in order to understand any of the components of managed care. The rapid growth and continued evolution of managed care has resulted in an ever-expanding and mutating set of definitions and operational structures. Although traditional terms such as *health maintenance organization* and *preferred provider organization* retain considerable utility, the terminology in this industry has an underlying instability. This characteristic should be looked upon not as a hindrance toward understanding but as a mark of the exciting and dynamic nature of the industry.

CHAPTER 3

Network Management and Reimbursement

LEARNING OBJECTIVES

- Understand the makeup of the health care delivery system network
- Understand the basic components of a physician network
- Understand the basic components of a hospital and ancillary services network
- Understand the basic reimbursement methods for physicians and hospitals

Managed care organizations (MCOs) such as health maintenance organizations (HMOs) or preferred provider organizations (PPOs) provide for the financing and delivery of health care services through networks of providers under contract. Certain types of MCOs, such as point-of-service (POS) plans and various types of service or indemnity insurance health plans, also provide financial coverage of some type for health care rendered by providers who are not under contract. Integrated delivery systems (IDSs) provide health care services under managed care, although they do not necessarily provide for the financing of those services.

77

The contracted provider networks are referred to collectively as the health care delivery system or simply as "the network." The network is composed principally of physicians, nonphysician professionals (e.g., psychologists), hospitals, providers of various ancillary services such as diagnostic services (e.g., radiology and laboratory services) and therapeutic services (e.g., physical therapy), and pharmacists, among others (Figure 3–1).

GENERAL CONTRACTING ISSUES

It is the presence of a contract at all that defines an MCO—if there are no contracts between the plan and a network of providers, then it is not an MCO but rather some type of indemnity insurance plan (Figure 3–2).

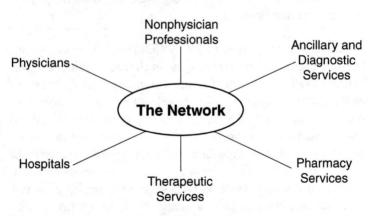

Figure 3–1 Components of a provider network.

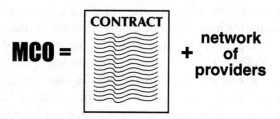

Figure 3–2 The new math.

Definitions

The contract must specify what it covers and what it does not cover. Items that require definition include the following:

- plan components such as member, subscriber, medical director, provider, payer, physician, and hospital
- routine medical services and experimental and/or investigational services
- "medically necessary" and "emergent or urgent" medical services
- services that providers are expected to provide under the contract
- services that providers are *not* expected to provide under the contract

Standard MCO Contract Provisions

Required Qualifications and Credentials

The contract must make it absolutely clear that the provider must have and maintain certain qualifications and credentials in order to remain under contract to the MCO. Common examples for physicians include an unrestricted license to practice medicine, hospital privileges (i.e., the right to admit patients), malpractice insurance, and board certification. Common examples for hospitals include certification by appropriate accreditation agencies, full participation in Medicare (and often Medicaid), and maintenance of licensure

Required Compliance with the MCO's Utilization and Quality Management Programs

The contract describes the management programs of the MCO that focus on resource utilization and quality of care. In addition, it describes the obligations of both the provider and the MCO under these programs.

"Hold Harmless" and "No Balance Billing" Clauses

A highly important section of the contract outlines the provider's agreement to accept as payment in full for medical services provided to MCO members the amount that the MCO determines to be appropriate. For example, if a physician normally charges $100 for an office visit but the MCO's fee schedule allows only $75, then the physician agrees that, under no circumstances, will he or she bill the member for the $25 difference; in other words, the provider will "hold the member harmless" from any additional payment. The provider agrees to accept payment only from the MCO, except for the portion that is the clear obligation of the member, such as a co-payment (e.g., a $10 per visit payment), coinsurance (e.g., 20 percent of the total *allowed* by the MCO, not the total originally billed by the provider), or a specified deductible (e.g., a

$200 amount that the member must pay for health care services before any insurance coverage begins to apply). The provision applies to hospitals in the same way.

This clause also prohibits the provider from billing the member even in the event that the MCO does not pay the fee at all (if, for example, the MCO refused to pay because the service was not authorized for coverage). All state and federal regulatory agencies require the "no balance billing" clause for contracts between providers and the MCO for almost all forms of MCOs. It is an absolute requirement in HMOs and a likely requirement for most PPOs and service plans as well (see Chapter 2).

Payment or Reimbursement Terms

The actual financial terms of a provider's contract with an MCO change periodically. Because it is far easier to change an appendix or attachment than to amend an entire contract, the reimbursement terms usually appear in an appendix or attachment to the contract.

Other-Party Liability: Subrogation and Coordination of Benefits

In some cases, there may be more than one payer responsible for coverage of medical services. For example, a man may have health insurance through work, while his wife also has health insurance through her own place of employment. If the couple's child receives medical care, which parent's insurance will be primarily responsible and which parent's insurance will be secondarily responsible (Figure 3–3)? Further, can both policies be used to increase the total amount of insur-

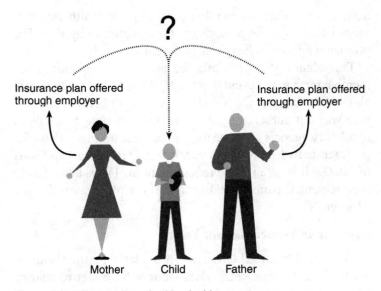

Figure 3–3 The question raised by dual insurance coverage.

ance coverage available? Similarly, which insurance will cover medical services provided to an MCO member if those services are the result of an accident (e.g., an automobile accident in which the auto insurance pays for part of the medical services)? The contract sets out the basic rules for dealing with such situations.

Term and Termination

One section of the contract specifies how long the contract is for and under what circumstances either party may terminate it. Termination provisions have become very complex in many states. In past decades, either party could terminate the contract simply by giving adequate notice (i.e., telling the other party as far ahead of time as the contract requires for such notification, such as 90 days). Recently, however, many states have begun to require MCOs that no longer want a provider's services to furnish the provider with the reasons for termination, and a few states have created due process requirements that allow a terminated provider to dispute the termination. No laws have been enacted that require providers to furnish reasons for wishing to terminate a contract with an MCO or that allow the MCO to dispute the termination.

There are three common categories of reasons for termination:

1. Inadequate quality of care. An MCO must take action to remove an incompetent provider from the network. Such terminations are reportable to the appropriate government agencies (e.g., the state department of licensure or health; the National Practitioner Data Bank).
2. Failure to meet recredentialing requirements. Providers may have a change in their professional status. For example, a physician may fail to requalify for board certification (requalification is required every 10 years in many specialties) or may have had his or her license restricted.
3. Business reasons. An MCO or a provider may conclude that having no contract is preferable to the terms of the existing contract. In the case of an MCO, the MCO's medical managers may have determined that a particular provider's practice behavior is unsuitable for a managed care environment. It is this third category that has cre-

ated great distress among providers and has led several states to pass laws that inhibit MCOs from terminating physicians for business reasons.

PHYSICIANS

In general, physicians are health care professionals who have a license to prescribe medications, privileges to admit patients to hospitals, and other related attributes. They most commonly have earned the degree of medical doctor (MD) or doctor of osteopathy (DO). In many states, and often by convention, other professionals, such as a doctor of chiropractic (DC), may also carry the designation of physician. This follows common usage in the managed care industry.

There are many ways to classify physicians. It is most common to differentiate physicians based on whether they are functioning in the role of primary care physician or specialty care physician. There is a third distinction that is really a variation of specialty care physician. This is a form of a specialty care physician organization that is highly focused on providing a particular type of health care. The distinctions between these types of physicians are not always clear. They remain useful, however, because many aspects of managed care are based on them.

Primary Care Physicians

In virtually all health care systems, care rendered by physicians in the specialties of family practice, internal medicine, and pediatrics is considered primary care. General practitioners (i.e., physicians who have not obtained full residency training beyond their internships) may also be considered PCPs, but few MCOs employ them—except in rural or underserved areas where there may not be a sufficient number of residency-trained PCPs to provide care to all MCO members.

Many OB/GYN specialists feel that they too deliver primary care to their patients. They argue that a young woman's gynecologist is often the only physician she sees for many years. This may be true in the case of generally healthy young women, but it is not always so for those who have medical problems that do not involve the female reproductive tract. Currently, almost all MCOs allow female members to have direct access to OB/GYNs. It should be noted that, in addition to simple market demands, many states have passed laws requiring MCOs to allow direct access to OB/GYNs. For clinical care that is beyond the scope of normal OB/GYN practice, the member must see the PCP for treatment or referral to another specialist.

Role of the Primary Care Physician

In all types of MCOs and IDSs, the PCP's role is extremely important. Many health care plans require enrollees to visit their PCP in order to obtain either direct care or a referral authorization for specialty care. Called a *gatekeeper* or *coordinating physician,* this PCP coordinates all services for the enrollees in the PCP's practice. Even when there is no such requirement, many U.S. citizens receive most of their regular health care from PCPs.

Although it is common for PCPs to be trained in primary care, there are certain clinical circumstances when it is better for a specialist to act as the PCP. For example (as discussed in Chapter 4), a patient with severe heart disease may be better managed by a cardiologist for all medical problems than by a general internist, since almost any clinical condition will have an impact on the heart in such a patient. A few MCOs use what they refer to as a "flexible gatekeeper," a specialty care physician that their members can choose to serve as their PCP. For example, a member may choose a cardiologist as his or her PCP because the cardiologist is also an internist. Even if the term *flexible gatekeeper* is not used, specialty-trained internists frequently function as PCPs. Some confusion may arise, however, if the same physician is functioning as a PCP for some members and a specialty care physician for others.

The number of PCPs that an MCO hires is based almost entirely on market demand and not on efficiency issues (i.e., the number hired is not necessarily the number able to serve the enrolled population most efficiently). For example, the typical group or staff model HMO may have one physician for every 1,200 to 1,500 members, but such figures are meaningless in any form of open-panel MCO. The market dictates that large numbers of PCPs in accessible locations are necessary for a successful open-panel MCO; small panels are less desirable to consumers and employers.

Nonphysician or Midlevel Practitioners in Primary Care

Among the nonphysician or midlevel practitioners in primary care are physician's assistants and nurse practitioners. There are several different types of nurse practitioner designations, each having a different focus and training; for example, there are advanced practice nurses, nurse-midwives, nurse-anesthetists, and clinical nurse specialists. The presence of such nonphysician practitioners is generally an asset in managed care because they are able to deliver excellent primary care, provide more health maintenance and health promotion services, and tend to spend more time with patients.

Nonphysician providers may play an especially important role in the management of chronically ill patients. They may coordinate care or function as case managers for patients with diseases such as chronic asthma, diabetes, and the like. In a similar vein, nonphysician providers may take a key role in managing the care of high-risk patients, using practice protocols for disease prevention and health maintenance in this population. Certified nurse-midwives may provide not only services for routine deliveries but also primary gynecological care using practice guidelines and protocols.

Specialty Care Physicians

Also commonly referred to as *specialists*, specialty care physicians (e.g., cardiologists, surgeons) provide specialty health care services, even if some of those services are essentially the same as those delivered by PCPs. In other words, in an MCO, a physician who is not a PCP will be considered a specialty care physician. As noted earlier, it is possible for a single physician to be both, although rarely for the same patient. For example, a cardiologist may be the PCP for an enrolled panel of members but also serve as a specialty care physician to other PCPs. This cardiologist cannot see a member as a PCP, however, and then refer the same member back to him- or herself as a specialty care physician (thus generating two bills).

It is becoming increasingly common for specialty care physicians to function as PCPs for those members with significant chronic illnesses, even if they do not otherwise function as PCPs. For example, through special arrangements with the MCO, a cardiologist may serve as the primary and coordinating physician for a patient with severe congestive heart failure.

"Carve-out" and Specialty Care Services

Not only specialty care physicians practicing individually or in medical groups but also specialty care organizations may provide specialty services. In these cases, the specialty care services focus on defined disease states or medical conditions. The specialty care organization may be a company, a large medical group, or a specialty independent practice association (IPA). For example, it is common for MCOs to contract with a company to provide all behavioral health and substance abuse services. Less commonly, an MCO may contract with an organization for all services related to renal dialysis or cancer care. This is often referred to as a "carve-out" service, in that the costs and mechanisms for managing the service have been carved out of the overall budget and medical management program and are handled separately.

Credentialing

An MCO has an obligation to verify that the physicians in its network meet the professional standards that it has established for its participating providers. The credentialing process actually begins before a physician receives a contract in the first place, and recredentialing takes place every two years.

The MCO often performs what is referred to as "primary source" credentialing, that is, obtaining documents directly from pertinent agencies or schools. The process of credentialing often varies little from MCO to MCO, however, and if each MCO conducts primary source credentialing individually, a significant burden is placed on the physicians and the MCO staff. Therefore, MCOs frequently rely on a third-party credentialing verification organization to perform primary credentialing on a physician. The credentialing verification organization must itself be certified by the appropriate certification agency.

The common basic elements of initial credentialing (i.e., the credentialing that occurs before a physician joins the network) include the following:

- training (copy of certificates)
  1. location of training
  2. type of training
- specialty care board eligibility or certification (copy of certificate)
- current state medical license (copy of certificate)
  1. restrictions
  2. history of loss of license in any state
- medical license numbers in all states where provider is licensed
- Drug Enforcement Agency (DEA) number and copy of certificate
- federal tax identification number

- Medicare, Medicaid, and other existing provider identification numbers (to be replaced by the National Provider Identifier some time in 2004 or 2005 under the provisions of the Health Insurance Portability and Accountability Act of 1996 [HIPAA])
- Social Security number
- hospital privileges
  1. names of hospitals
  2. scope of practice privileges
- malpractice insurance
  1. name of insurance carrier
  2. currency of coverage (copy of face sheet)
  3. scope of coverage (i.e., financial limits and procedures covered)
- malpractice history
  1. pending claims
  2. successful claims against the physician, either judged or settled
- location and telephone numbers of all offices
- yes/no questions regarding:
  1. limitations or suspensions of privileges
  2. suspension from participation in any government programs
  3. suspension or restriction of DEA license
  4. cancellation of malpractice insurance
  5. felony conviction
  6. drug or alcohol abuse
  7. chronic or debilitating illnesses

Additional elements of initial credentialing that are not always required include

- hours of operation
- provisions for emergency care and backup
- use of midlevel practitioners (e.g., physician's assistants or clinical nurse practitioners)
- in-office surgery capabilities
- in-office testing capabilities
- languages spoken
- work history, at least over the past five years
- areas of special medical interest
- continuing medical education

The MCO obtains the credentialing information from the physician, from a credentialing verification organization, or directly from the relevant agencies (e.g., the physician's medical school). In addition, the MCO (as well as all hospitals) must query the National Practitioner Data Bank (NPDB). Created under the Health Care Quality Improvement Act of 1986 (HCQIA), with final regulations published in 1989 (*Federal Register* 45 C.F.R. Part 60), the NPDB serves as a central repository of information on the following topics:

- malpractice payments made for the benefit of physicians, dentists, and other health care practitioners
- licensure actions taken by state medical boards and state boards of dentistry against physicians and dentists and other health care practitioners who are licensed or otherwise authorized by a state to provide health care services
- actions taken as a result of professional reviews, primarily against physicians and dentists by hospitals and other health care entities, including HMOs, group practices, and professional societies

- actions taken by the Drug Enforcement Agency
- Medicare/Medicaid participation exclusions

Information reported to the NPDB is considered confidential and may not be disclosed except as specified in the final regulations. The enabling act, HCQIA, also provides for qualified immunity from antitrust lawsuits for credentialing activities, as well as professional medical staff sanctions, when the terms of the act are followed.

More recently, the Healthcare Integrity and Protection Data Bank (HIPDB) was created under HIPAA to combat fraud and abuse in health insurance and health care delivery. The HIPDB is a national data collection program for the reporting and disclosure of certain final adverse actions taken against health care providers, suppliers, and practitioners (excluding settlements in which no findings of liability have been made). It is to contain information about

- civil judgments against health care providers, suppliers, or practitioners in federal or state courts related to the delivery of health care items or services
- federal or state criminal convictions against health care providers, suppliers, or practitioners related to the delivery of health care items or services
- actions by federal or state agencies responsible for the licensing and certification of health care providers, suppliers, or practitioners
- exclusion of health care providers, suppliers, or practitioners from participation in federal or state health care programs

- any other adjudicated actions or decisions that the secretary of the Department of Health and Human Services establishes through regulations.

After the physician becomes part of the network, recredentialing occurs every two years. The credentialing information may be simply updated by the physician directly or through the credentialing verification organization. At the time of recredentialing, many MCOs add information gleaned from quality assurance surveys and member satisfaction surveys. It is also necessary to requery the NPDB and the HIPDB.

The basic elements of recredentialing include the following:

- current status of state medical license (copy of current valid certificate)
  1. restrictions
  2. history of loss of license in any state
- copy of current valid DEA certificate
- any changes to Medicare, Medicaid, or other existing provider identification numbers (to be replaced by the National Provider Identifier some time in 2004 or 2005 under the provisions of HIPAA)
- status of hospital privileges
  1. names of hospitals
  2. scope of practice privileges
- current malpractice insurance status
  1. name of insurance carrier
  2. currency of coverage (copy of face sheet)
  3. scope of coverage (financial limits and procedures covered)

- malpractice history over past two years
  1. pending claims
  2. successful claims against the physician, either judged or settled
- yes/no questions regarding
  1. limitations or suspensions of privileges
  2. suspension from government programs
  3. suspension or restriction of DEA license
  4. cancellation of malpractice insurance
  5. felony conviction
  6. drug or alcohol abuse
  7. chronic or debilitating illnesses

Reimbursement of Physicians

Managed care organizations frequently pay their physicians, especially PCPs, according to some form of performance- or risk-based reimbursement system (i.e., reimbursement has some element of risk for medical expenses). Less commonly, specialty care physicians may receive payment for their services under some form of risk-based reimbursement.

The compensation of physicians working under direct contract to MCOs rather than providing services through an intermediary differs from the compensation of individual physicians in organized groups, staff models, or IDSs. It is possible and even common to use these methods of reimbursement for an individual physician in such groups. For example, a medical group might blend the three basic forms of compensation—capitation, fee-for-service, and salary—to pay individual physicians no matter how the group itself receives payment.

The objective of any reimbursement system is to better align the compensation of physicians with the overall goals of managed care. By itself, it is unlikely that any compensation system will have much of an impact, however. A reimbursement system is simply one of the many tools available in managed care and will probably fail to achieve the desired goals in the absence of other vital tools, such as competent management of utilization and quality. Although there are few basic ways of reimbursing physicians and other professionals, there are countless variations on themes and numerous combinations. In addition, withholds or risk and incentive compensation may be applied to any method or combination of methods.

Managed care is marked by a high degree of change and variation. Change is produced by market forces, new managed care practices, new laws and regulations (especially in Medicare and Medicaid), and uncountable other factors (Figure 3–4). As a result, provider types and the reimbursement mechanisms are rarely found in their pure form.

Capitation

Although the fee-for-service system remains the most common form of physician reimbursement, capitation is a powerful and popular option for managed care. It involves fixed payments made on a per member per month (PMPM) basis regardless of the use of services. In other words, the physician receives a fixed amount of money each month for every member of the MCO who enrolls in that physician's panel of patients. Whether the member seeks care every day or never seeks care at all, the amount of money that the physician receives does not vary.

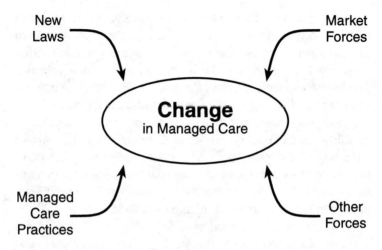

Figure 3–4 Change factors affecting managed care.

The actual capitation fees are usually adjusted based on the age and sex of each enrolled member, because there is some correlation between those factors and utilization (i.e., medical costs). In general, older members use more health care services than younger members, and young women use more services than young men. Capitation fees, in rare cases, are adjusted based on other factors, such as geographic location.

The key to making capitation work is received fees from a large number of members most of whom will not need extensive (and expensive) services. Because the members of an HMO must select a single PCP to provide and coordinate care, ensuring that they are counted only once, capitation is most easily applied to PCPs in HMOs. In fact, well over half of open-panel HMOs use capitation for reimbursing PCPs. Capitation may be used for physicians in high-volume specialties as well, but for specialists there must be some mechanism to ensure that, except in special circumstances, the members for whom the HMO is making capitation payments will not seek or receive services from noncapitated providers.

Capitation payments made directly to providers may be subject to a withhold. For example, the MCO may hold back 10 percent of the total amount of capitation to be paid to a provider in order to cover unexpectedly high rates of utilization. Withholds are less common than they once were, as many MCOs now prefer to base their programs primarily on incentives rather than penalties.

Incentive payments are common in MCOs, at least for PCPs. In general, the incentive payment is a reward for providers who keep down utilization or medical costs, although incentive payments based on high-quality care, accessibility, and member satisfaction are becoming more common. In a typical arrangement, a pool of money is set aside in an amount determined by the number of members. The MCO applies the money during the year against expenses in a defined category, such as referral or hospital costs, and then distributes the remainder at the end of the year (in part or in whole) to the physicians based on utilization patterns, either of the entire panel of physicians or of each individual physician.

The variations on the theme of capitation are numerous (Figure 3–5). For example, although used infrequently, contact capitation is sometimes used to reimburse specialty care physicians. In this system, patients choose specialists of the kind they need to see, and the MCO then pays each specialist a

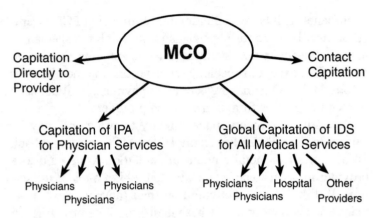

Figure 3–5 Examples of types of capitation.

percentage of the total capitation dollars that the MCO had set aside to cover the care that its members might need from such a specialist. For example, if 100 members received orthopedic care from six orthopedists, then the MCO would distribute the total capitation dollars to those orthopedists based on the percentage of the 100 members that each orthopedist saw (e.g., if one saw 15 members, that orthopedist would receive 15 percent of the total amount available for orthopedic care). Adjustments are also made for severity of illness, duration of the episode of care, and other variables, increasing the complexity of the system. Contact capitation requires very large membership bases and highly sophisticated computer systems.

Global capitation differs from ordinary capitation in that the provider receiving the capitation payment under global capitation may not be the provider actually delivering the health care services. In a global capitation system, the MCO covers all or most medical costs through capitation payments to a large, organized medical group or an IDS—rarely, if ever, to individual physicians or small medical groups. The large group receives capitation payments that cover all the services it provides as well as any costs from services provided from outside the group. In other words, the globally capitated medical group is responsible for all the medical costs of the MCO members. This form of reimbursement is manageable only by very large groups or IDSs, and even then its track record has been very poor; many such groups have failed because of their inability to manage the risk for medical costs.

It is common for an IPA to receive global capitation payments on behalf of all the physicians in the IPA, even if the IPA does not, in turn, make global capitation payments to the individual providers or medical groups. In fact, it is the business of most IPAs to accept capitation payments for the entire network and then apply the more common forms of reimbursement (i.e., individual capitation or fee-for-service) to compensate individual physicians within the IPA. In the same way, certain group model HMOs use global capitation to reimburse the medical group for medical costs, even though the medical group itself pays individual physicians via salary.

Fee-for-Service

While remaining a significant form of reimbursement in HMOs, fee-for-service is nearly the only form of reimbursement in PPOs, service plans, and indemnity plans. Even HMOs that use a capitation system for PCPs usually reimburse referral specialists on a fee-for-service basis. In POS plans, it is difficult, if not impossible, to predict actual in-network utilization for each member, making capitation an unsuitable form of compensation for providers. Consequently, many of these plans reimburse even PCPs on a fee-for-service basis. Although somewhat less conducive to managed care than is capitation, fees for service are not necessarily unsuitable for managed care.

If not managed properly, a fee-for-service system can lead to higher costs than would occur under capitation. Therefore, it is common for HMOs that use a fee-for-service system to place the fees at some form of risk for the provider. A withhold on a percentage of the fees is the most common mechanism as discussed under the topic of capitation. If utilization exceeds that anticipated in the budget, the MCO uses the withhold to cover the cost overage; if utilization is below that anticipated, the withhold is paid out to providers (or at least those providers who have lower than budgeted medical costs). Some MCOs reduce fees if utilization becomes excessive. Other MCOs have experimented with global fees (i.e., a single fee for a visit or procedure regardless of how much or how little care the patient receives during that visit); this approach has had some success in preventing cost increases resulting from the use of fee codes that pay more.

The methods used to determine what fees to pay for each procedure or visit vary from MCO to MCO. In the past, MCOs often determined fees based on the "usual, customary, or reasonable" fees for services in that area, but over the past two decades this method became synonymous with uncontrolled fee inflation. Therefore, all MCOs now use some form of fee schedule, setting a maximum amount that a physician will be paid for each individual procedure or service. Physicians under contract to an MCO agree to accept the established amount as payment in full (except for any co-payment or coinsurance that the member must pay) and not charge the member the difference between the established amount and what the physicians normally ask.

The use of a relative value scale (RVS) to determine fees is quite common. The MCO assigns a value to each procedure or visit code and determines the fee by multiplying a set dollar amount against the relative value. For example, a procedure may have a relative value of 4.5, and the fee is calculated by multiplying $10 by 4.5, resulting in a fee of $45. (These numbers are for illustration purposes only and do not represent actual relative values or monetary multipliers.)

The most common type of RVS is the resource-based relative value scale (RBRVS) developed by the Health Care Financing Administration (now the Centers for Medicare & Medicaid Services, or CMS) for use in the Medicare program. Before the development of the RBRVS, most fee schedules and even routine RVSs were based on historical charge patterns, in which the fees for surgical and procedural services were higher than the fees for so-called cognitive services. For example, 20 minutes of surgery might generate a fee of $800, while 20 minutes of time with an internist in the office might generate a fee of $45. The RBRVS was created to address this imbalance by lowering the relative values of many procedural services and raising the relative values of many cognitive services. Although procedures still generate substantially higher fees than do cognitive services, some of the disparity has been reduced. Many MCOs simply adopt the RBRVS as CMS issues and updates it and then use it to calculate provider fees (though the monetary multipliers used differ among the MCOs).

Salary

Payment of a salary is the predominant method of physician reimbursement in closed-panel plans as well as in some group practices or situations where physicians are employees (e.g., full-time faculty, government-employed physicians, or some full-time hospital-based physicians). The employer may apply withholds to the physician's base salary, and incentive plans are common. In a withhold program, the employer holds back a small percentage of the salary (e.g., 10 percent). If medical costs exceed those anticipated, the employer uses the withheld amount to help cover the increased costs. If medical costs are as expected or below, the physician receives the withheld amount.

An incentive program is similar but may encompass more than measurements of medical costs. For example, an MCO or IDS may have a program in which it is possible for employed physicians to receive a bonus of as much as 10 percent to 20 percent of their base salary if they keep medical costs within anticipated limits, make every effort to ensure patient satisfaction, are very productive, comply with quality management programs, and fulfill other requirements established by the MCO or IDS. Incentive programs are more common than withhold programs, though in fact the difference may be more a question of wording than of functioning.

Stop-Loss Protection

It is in the interest of both the MCO and the physicians to prevent one or two very costly cases from inflicting a financial penalty on an individual physician. Therefore, in most cases of risk-based reimbursement, there is a limit on a physician's exposure to financial risk. Reaching that limit activates the physician's stop-loss protection. Such protection may be as simple as limiting any financial risk to the amount of the with-hold, if one exists. In other cases, such as where global capita-tion is involved, the degree of risk can be significantly higher (involving large sums of money) and may require the pur-chase of special insurance, sometimes referred to as stop-loss insurance or reinsurance.

In general, *stop-loss* means that at some point the amount of costs generated no longer are used to measure the performance or determine the reimbursement of a physician. Specific stop-loss protection shields the physician from high medical costs result-ing from an individual patient's case, while aggregate stop-loss protection shields the physician from a high total cost for the physician's entire panel of patients. The aim of both types of stop-loss protection is the same: to prevent high costs associated with untypical cases from having an adverse effect on the physician's reimbursement.

Legislation and Regulation Applicable to Physician Incentive Programs

In recent years, the federal government and many state gov-ernments have passed laws and created regulations that affect physician incentive programs. These apply primarily to capita-tion programs and to incentive programs that increase the income of a physician who provides fewer services. (Of course, there are no such regulations placed upon fee-for-service systems, as they reward physicians for doing more, not less, and the provision of more care is supposedly less likely to harm patients.)

Not all states have passed laws and promulgated regulations that apply to physician compensation and incentives under managed care. The laws and regulations that are in force show little consistency from one state to another. In general, state laws focus on the disclosure of financial incentives.

CMS has implemented regulations that place limits on physician incentive programs in Medicare and Medicaid MCOs. In general, these regulations outline a set of conditions that may be considered to place a physician at "significant financial risk," conditions that vary based on several factors (e.g., the size of the medical group at risk for medical costs, the percentage of total compensation at risk for medical costs). If there is a significant financial risk, then the MCO must provide specific levels and types of stop-loss insurance and may need to undertake special types of consumer satisfaction surveys. In addition, the federal regulations require disclosure of each physician's amount and type of financial risk, at least in the case of physicians providing care for Medicare and/or Medicaid patients.

HOSPITALS AND INSTITUTIONS

Obviously, an MCO needs for there to be hospitals and institutional providers in its service area (e.g., acute care hospitals, skilled and intermediate care facilities, and all types of ambulatory facilities). Every MCO must ensure that all its members have access to reasonably convenient acute care, especially emergency care. The licensure body for MCOs, often the state department of insurance, usually has requirements for the maximum permissible amount of time or distance that a member must travel in order to receive care; for example, it is common to require a drive time of 30 minutes or less to access an acute care hospital and emergency department. If an MCO is unable to provide access to a contracted facility within those time or distance limits, the state may refuse to license the MCO or at the least not allow the MCO to market services in any geographic area in which access to services is inadequate. Employers or purchasers may have similar or even stricter requirements for access.

Access is also a function of the services provided. For example, two nearby hospitals may differ in the services they offer; only one of the two may offer obstetric services, while the other might be the sole provider of trauma services. An MCO must take the types of services into account, as well as location, when building its network of providers.

The types of institutional providers that MCO members must have access to include subacute care facilities, rehabilitation centers, skilled and intermediate care facilities, and ambulatory facilities. Skilled and intermediate care facilities, often referred to as "nursing homes," play an important role in the Medicare and Medicaid programs and also have a place in commercial programs. Ambulatory surgical centers, or outpatient surgery centers, may be part of a hospital, may be owned by a hospital, or may be free-standing. Location is less important for these facilities, since virtually all care is elective, and therefore access to them is not urgent. Specific coverage for nonacute care varies from plan to plan.

Reimbursement Methods

There are a number of reimbursement methods available to MCOs in contracting with hospitals and other health care institutions (except in those few states where regulations diminish or prohibit creativity), and it is common to find an MCO using more than one method to reimburse a single institution. Exhibit 3–1 describes the various types of reimbursement methods.

Straight Charges

The simplest payment method in health care is to pay straight charges (i.e., charges undiscounted in any way). It is also obviously the most expensive. An MCO will agree to pay straight charges only in the event that it is unable to obtain any form of discount but wants to have a contract with a "no balance billing" clause in it to meet reserve and licensure requirements.

Exhibit 3–1 Reimbursement Methods

Straight Charges
Discount on Charges
   Straight discount on charges
   Sliding scale discount on charges
Per Diem Charges
   Straight per diem charges
   Sliding scale per diem
   Differential by day in hospital
Diagnosis-Related Groups
Case Rates and Package Pricing
Capitation or Percentage of Revenue
Contact Capitation
Periodic Interim Payments and Cash Advances
Package Pricing or Bundled Charges

Discount on Charges

Straight Discount on Charges. Another possible method is to discount charges by a straight percentage. In this method, the hospital submits its bill in the full amount, and the MCO discounts it by the previously agreed percentage and then pays it. The hospital accepts this payment as payment in full. The amount of discount that can be obtained will depend on the factors discussed earlier, such as the degree of competitiveness in the market, the desire of the hospital to receive patients from the MCO, and so forth. The straight discount method is common in markets with low levels of managed care penetration but is very uncommon in markets with high levels of managed care penetration.

Sliding Scale Discount on Charges. In markets with few MCOs but some level of competitiveness between hospitals, sliding scale discounts are an option. With a sliding scale, the percentage discount reflects the total volume of services provided. For example, there may be a 20-percent reduction in charges for 0 to 200 total bed days per year, with incremental increases in the discount as the number of bed days increases—up to a maximum percentage. An interim percentage discount is usually negotiated, and the parties reconcile at the end of the year based on the final total volume.

Whether to lump admissions and outpatient procedures together or deal with them separately is not as important as making sure that the parties deal with them both. With the rapidly climbing cost of outpatient care, an unanticipated overrun in outpatient charges could erase the savings obtained from a reduction of inpatient utilization.

Per Diem Charges

Straight Per Diem Charges. The most common type of arrangement is for MCOs to reimburse hospitals on the basis of straight per diem charges. The MCO negotiates a single per diem rate of payment per day in the hospital and pays that rate regardless of any actual charges or costs incurred. The per diem is simply an estimate of the charges or costs for an average day in that hospital minus the level of discount. The key to making a per diem work is predictability. If the MCO and hospital can accurately predict the number and mix of cases, then they can calculate an adequate per diem.

Hospital administrators are often reluctant to include days in the intensive care or obstetric units as part of the base per diem unless there is sufficient volume of regular medical-surgical cases to make the ultimate cost predictable. For a small MCO or one that is not limiting the number of participating hospitals, administrators may be concerned that the MCO will use their hospital for expensive cases at a low per diem while they use competing hospitals for less costly cases. In this situation, a good option is to negotiate multiple sets of per diem charges based on service type (e.g., medical-surgical procedures, obstetrics, intensive care, neonatal intensive care, and rehabilitation) or a combination of per diems and a flat case rate for obstetrics (costs are predictable for routine obstetric care and a flat case rate incents the hospital toward efficiency).

Some MCOs may also negotiate an agreement by which they reimburse the hospital for certain expensive surgical implants provided at the hospital's actual cost of the implant. Such reimbursement would be limited to a defined list of implants (e.g., inner ear implants) for which the cost to the hospital for the implant is far greater than is recoverable under the per diem arrangement.

Sliding Scale Per Diem. Like the sliding scale discount on charges, the sliding scale per diem is based on total volume. In this case, the MCO agrees to pay an interim per diem for each day that one of its members spends in the hospital during the year. The more days that the MCO members spend in the hospital during the year, however, the lower the per diem rate. Depending on the total number of bed days or admissions in the year, the MCO will either pay a lump sum settlement at the end of the year or withhold an amount from the final payment to adjust for the actual number of bed days or admissions. It is wise to review and possibly adjust the interim per diem on a quarterly or semiannual basis so as to reduce disparities caused by unexpected changes in utilization patterns.

Differential by Day in Hospital. Most hospitalizations are more expensive on the first day. For example, the first day charges for surgical cases include operating suite costs, the operating surgical team costs (nurses and recovery), and so forth. The reimbursement method for such services is generally a variation of the per diem approach, with the first day paid at a higher rate.

Diagnosis-Related Groups

MCOs often use diagnosis-related groups (DRGs) for the purpose of reimburseing hospitals. There are publications that contain information on DRG categories, criteria, outliers (cases that may fall into a DRG category, but are far more severe and require far longer lengths of stay than the DRG covers), and trim points (the cost or length of stay that triggers supplementation or replacement of the DRG payment by another payment mechanism; applied to outliers) to enable MCOs to negotiate DRG payment methods based on Medicare rates or, in some cases, state-regulated rates. Currently, as used by CMS for Medicare, DRGs are not severity adjusted.

Case Rates and Package Pricing

Whatever mechanism an MCO uses for hospital reimbursement, it may still be necessary to address certain categories of procedures or services and negotiate special rates for those categories. In the area of obstetrics, for example, it is common for an MCO either to negotiate a case rate for a normal vaginal delivery and a case rate for a cesarean section or to negotiate a blended rate for both. In the case of blended case rates (which are much preferred over separate rates for the two types of deliveries because they eliminate any financial incentive to do cesarean sections), the expected reimbursement for each type of delivery is multiplied by the expected (or desired) percentage of utilization. For example, a case rate for vaginal delivery may be $3,500; for cesarean section, $4,500. If utilization is expected to be 80 percent vaginal delivery and 20 percent cesarean section, the blended case rate would be $3,700 ($3,500 $\times$ 0.8 = $2,800; $4,500 $\times$ 0.2 = $900; $2,800 + $900 = $3,700). Other common areas in which case rates make sense are procedures at tertiary (i.e., specialty) hospitals; for example, MCOs may establish case rates for coronary artery bypass surgery, heart transplants, or certain types of cancer treatment.

These procedures, although relatively infrequent, are tremendously costly.

Package pricing or bundled case rates are all-inclusive rates paid for both institutional and professional services. The MCO negotiates a flat rate for a procedure (e.g., coronary artery bypass surgery), and that rate covers the fees of all parties who provide services connected with that procedure, including preadmission and postdischarge care. Bundled case rates are not uncommon in teaching facilities, where the faculty members practice as part of the hospital staff and are used to sharing income with the teaching hospital.

Capitation or Percentage of Revenue

As it does with physicians, a capitation plan may provide for reimbursement of a hospital or institution on a PMPM basis to cover all the facility's costs in providing medical care for a defined population of members. The payment may be varied according to the age and sex of patients but does not fluctuate with premium revenue. A percentage of revenue plan, on the other hand, involves paying a fixed percentage of premium revenue (i.e., a percentage of the collected premium payments) to the hospital or institution, again to cover all its services. The difference between capitation and percentage of revenue is that the percentage of revenue may vary with the premium rate charged and the actual revenue collected, while capitation is a fixed amount of reimbursement—it remains the same regardless of how much or how little the MCO collects in premium revenue.

In both methods, the hospital or institution stands the entire risk for the cost of any services that it provides for the defined membership base; if the hospital cannot provide the services itself, the cost for such care is deducted from the capitation payment. For this type of arrangement to be successful, a hospital must know that it will be serving a clearly defined segment of an MCO's enrolled population and that it will be able to provide most of the services that those members will need. In these plans, the PCP is clearly associated with just one hospital. Alternatively, if the MCO is dealing with a multihospital system with multiple facilities in the MCO's service area, it may be reasonable to expect that the hospitals in the system can care for the MCO's members on an exclusive basis.

It is necessary to clearly define what is covered under the capitation plan and what is not covered. For example, the capitation plan may include outpatient procedures, but the MCO and hospital need to account for outpatient procedures that are performed outside of the hospital's service area. Will home health care be part of the capitation plan, and if so, what agency is to provide that service? It is unwise to place the hospital at risk for services that it cannot control.

Capitation dramatically improves cash flow to the hospital (as it is prepayment for services), makes revenue predictable, and results in profits if utilization is well managed. In the recent past, however, some hospitals have simply not been able to manage the financial risk associated with capitation plans because they lack the financial management tools and expertise, utilization management skills, and information management capabilities to manage the risks associated with a broad population of members. When the membership base of capitated lives is small, then chance becomes as important as clinical management or even more so. As a result, many hospitals that once sought out capitation are now declining to participate in capitation programs.

Contact Capitation

Like contact capitation for the reimbursement of specialty physicians, contact capitation for the reimbursement of hospitals and other institutions is not common. In brief, capitation under this type of plan is tied to the percentage of the MCO members admitted to a hospital, with adjustments for the type of service. For example, suppose the capitation rate is $40 PMPM. The MCO has 100,000 members, and 50 percent of admissions go to a particular hospital that month. The payment to that hospital, therefore, is $2,000,000 ($40 × (100,000 × 0.5) = $2,000,000). It is usually necessary to make adjustments for service type, however, as well as for severity of illness. Such adjustments can quickly become complicated. For example, if three hospitals all provide cardiac services, two of them perform heart catheterizations and basic heart surgery, but only one provides advanced cardiac interventions, then trying to allocate costs based on severity becomes a nightmare.

Again like contact capitation for the reimbursement of specialty physicians, contact capitation agreements with institutions require sophisticated information systems, more sophisticated than the information systems possessed by some MCOs. However, in contrast, the number of participating institutions is generally lower than the number of specialist physicians in a network, which theoretically makes contact capitation agreements with institutions more manageable.

Contact capitation can be combined with case rates or other capitation rates. Obstetric care is often carved out and reimbursed using another reimbursement method, such as case rates, or through a separate capitation program.

Periodic Interim Payments and Cash Advances

It was once common but now is rare for an MCO to make periodic interim payments (PIPs) or a cash advance to a hospital in order to cover expected claims. A PIP is a regular cash payment made to the hospital, with actual expenses being deducted from the PIP on an ongoing (e.g., monthly) basis; the cash advance is similar, but may not be quite as regular. The cash advance is periodically replenished if it falls below a certain amount. Hospitals may receive payment for services provided directly from the cash advance, or the MCO may pay claims outside it, in which case the cash advance serves as an advance deposit. The value of this approach to a hospital is that it ensures a positive cash flow. In fact, PIPs and cash advances are so valuable to a hospital that they may generate a discount by themselves.

This mechanism is particularly effective in those periods when an unusually high number of claims is overwhelming an MCO's payment system or the MCO is otherwise unable to process payments in a timely manner. The cash advance allows the MCO to meet timely payment provisions and keeps the hospital financially sound while allowing additional time for the MCO to resolve problems with its payment systems.

Outpatient Procedures

As mentioned earlier, the shift from inpatient to outpatient care has not gone unnoticed by hospital administrators. As care has shifted, so have charges. Outpatient charges can often exceed the cost of an inpatient day unless steps are taken to address the imbalance.

Because most emergency services do not result in a hospital admission, these services are often considered a form of outpatient care. It is common for MCOs to include the costs of emergency department services in their reimbursement methodologies for inpatient care when the services do result in an admission. When emergency department services do not result in an admission, however, reimbursement usually falls along the same lines as those for other outpatient services.

Although emergency department services are often a form of convenience care (i.e., patients seek care during nonstandard hours for medical problems that are not necessarily emergencies), the primary reason for emergency departments remains the provision of care for true emergencies. Because the level of care required for true emergencies can vary widely, depending on the severity of the problem, some hospitals will not contract for emergency department services under the same terms as elective outpatient care. The differences in terms require careful negotiation between the MCO and the hospital.

Discounts on Charges

Either straight discounts or sliding scale discounts may be applied to outpatient charges. Some hospital administrators argue that the cost of delivering highly technical outpatient care actually is greater than the average per diem cost of inpatient care, primarily because the per diem cost is based on more than a single day in the hospital, which spreads the costs over a greater number of reimbursable days. Some MCOs have responded by simply admitting patients to the hospital for their outpatient surgery, paying the per diem, and sending the patients home. Many MCOs negotiate a clause in their contracts with hospitals to ensure that the cost of outpatient surgery never exceeds the cost of an inpatient day, whereas other MCOs concede the problem of front-loading (i.e., for an inpatient stay, all the costs occur right up front; the lower costs of the recovery days balance out the higher cost of the first day when the procedure occurred) surgical services and agree to pay outpatient charges at a fixed percentage of the per diem (e.g., 125 percent of the average per diem).

Package Pricing or Bundled Charges

With package pricing or bundled charges for outpatient procedures, MCOs bundle all the various charges (e.g., the cost of supplies, the room where the procedure took place, medications, nursing support, recovery room costs, discharge activities, and so forth) into one single charge. They may use their own data to develop the bundled charges or use outside data such as those available from a national actuarial firm. Bundled charges are generally tied to a principal procedure code used by the facility. Bundled charges may be added together in the event that more than one procedure is performed, although the second procedure is discounted because the patient was already in the facility and using services.

Related to the use of bundled charges is the establishment of tiered rates. In this approach, the outpatient department categorizes all procedures into several categories. The MCO then pays a different rate for each category, but that rate covers all services performed in the outpatient department, and only one category is used at a time (i.e., the hospital cannot add several categories together for a single patient encounter).

Ambulatory Visits

In the reimbursement of ambulatory visits or encounters, there are two classification systems: ambulatory patient groups (APGs) and ambulatory payment classifications (APCs). Both are in the public domain. A variety of payers (e.g., Medicaid and several Blue Cross/Blue Shield plans) were already using APGs prior to the introduction of APCs. Beginning in 2000, HCFA began implementing APCs for outpatient prospective payment in hospital outpatient departments and ambulatory surgery centers for Medicare patients. Because of this, APCs are fast becoming the package pricing system of choice for MCOs.

Although APGs and APCs are based on procedures rather than simply on diagnoses, contain a greater degree of adjustment for severity, and are considerably more complex, they are to outpatient services what DRGs are to inpatient services. If more than one procedure is performed, the MCO will receive claims for each, but there is significant discounting for the additional charges.

Ancillary Services

The collection of services that are provided as an adjunct to basic primary or specialty services are called ancillary services. They include almost everything other than institutional services (although institutions can provide ancillary services).

Ancillary services may be diagnostic or therapeutic. Ancillary diagnostic services include laboratory, radiology, nuclear testing, computed tomography (CT), magnetic resonance imaging (MRI), electroencephalography, and cardiac testing. Ancillary therapeutic services include cardiac rehabilitation, noncardiac rehabilitation, physical therapy, occupational therapy, and speech therapy.

Pharmacy services are ancillary services that account for significant costs and have been subject to recent price and usage inflation. An MCO may consider mental health and substance abuse services to be ancillary, but they are really core services. Emergency services, sometimes considered ancillary as well, are also actually core medical services.

Because most ancillary services require an order from a physician, the cost of such services is dependent on the utilization patterns of physicians. To reduce the cost of ancillary services, it is necessary to change these patterns (see Chapter 4). The other primary method of controlling the cost of ancillary services is to contract for such services in a way that makes the cost predictable. In fact, many MCOs rely far more heavily on favorable contracting terms to manage the cost of these services than they do on managing utilization.

Contracting and Reimbursement for Diagnostic and Therapeutic Ancillary Services

The development of a contracting and reimbursement system for ancillary services is one of the first and most important steps that an MCO can take in dealing with costs in this area. Many ancillary services are among the first to be carved out of the main medical delivery system and assigned to another organization able to accept the risks and responsibilities of providing such services, achieve economies of scale, and manage the overall cost and quality of the services.

Closed-panel HMOs, large medical groups, and IDSs have the option of providing certain ancillary services in-house. Management must conduct a cost-benefit analysis to determine whether that is a better course of action than contracting with an outside provider. Managing utilization is no less difficult when the service is in-house, however, because there is often a perception that referral for that service is free and certainly convenient.

Open-panel and closed-panel MCOs that do not have ancillary services in-house must contract for the services. An MCO usually has its choice of hospital-based services (sometimes these are the only option), free-standing (independent) services, or office-based services. A combination of such factors as quality, cost, access, service (e.g., turnaround time for testing), and convenience for members determines the choice. Unlike the physicians who provide medical services, the set of providers of a particular ancillary service usually make up a small percentage of the total number of providers. This allows the MCO to have greater leverage in negotiating with these providers as well as greater control over the quality of the services themselves.

In HMOs or MCOs that have absolute limitations on benefits for ancillary services, a capitation approach is often effective. To establish a capitated reimbursement system for ancillary services, it is necessary to calculate the expected frequency of need for the service and the expected or desired cost, and then spread this amount over the membership base on a monthly basis. The MCOs that allow significant benefits for out-of-network use (e.g., POS plans) may still use a capitation system, but only for the in-network costs; they must pay out-of-network costs through the regular fee allowances. If the capitated provider limits access strictly or cannot meet demand, the MCO will end up paying twice—once through capitation and a second time through fee-for-service. If the MCO has a large membership base, it may be possible to forecast cost and usage even under a POS plan, but if the MCO has a small enrollment base, capitation for benefit plans other than a pure HMO plan may not be feasible. This is because with a small enrollment base, the effects of random chance (e.g., the number of severe auto accidents) is higher than the effect of valid statistics (e.g., the number of auto accidents that can be expected for every 500,000 people).

Though this would be unusual, a POS plan may have no out-of-network benefits for some ancillary services, making it easier to establish a capitation system (i.e., since the POS does not offer out-of-network ancillary services, it does not need to try and adjust for in-network vs. out-of-network differences in cost). Simple PPOs generally are unable to use capitation because they are unable to adjust for in-network uses vs. out-of-network use for any specific provider and must depend on fee allowances or other forms of episode-related reimbursement.

Not all types of ancillary services lend themselves to capitation. If an ancillary service is highly self-contained, then it is easier to use a capitation system; for example, physical therapy usually is limited to treatment given by physical therapists and does not involve other types of ancillary service providers. Home health care, on the other hand, often involves home health care nurses and clinical aides, durable medical equipment, home infusion and medication supplies and equipment, home physical therapy, and so forth.

A number of MCOs have successfully used capitation for home health care services, although those have tended to be larger MCOs with sufficient volume to permit the accurate prediction of costs in all of these different areas. Other MCOs have been able to use this approach successfully only for parts of home health care (e.g., home respiratory therapy). In other areas, a combination of capitation and fixed case rates (e.g., for a course of chemotherapy) may be successful.

A recent variant on capitation is similar to the single specialty management organization or specialty network manager discussed earlier. In this case, a single entity accepts capitation from the MCO for all of the providers of a particular ancillary service (e.g., physical therapy). That organization then serves as a network manager or even as an IPA. The participating ancillary service providers may be subcontractors to the network manager and may receive payment either through subcapitation or through a form of fee-for-service. In all events, the network manager is at risk for the total costs of the capitated service even though the participating ancillary service providers are usually at risk as well through capitation, fee adjustments, withholds, and so forth.

Managed care organizations that do not have the option of capitation may still achieve considerable savings from discounts. Diagnostic ancillary services are often high-volume services, so it is usually not difficult to obtain reasonable discounts or to negotiate a fee schedule. Therapeutic ancillary service providers may be willing to accept case rates or tiered case rates. In this form of reimbursement, the ancillary service provider receives a fixed amount for a particular case regardless of the number of visits or resources used in providing services. For home health care involving high-intensity services such as chemotherapy or other high-technology services, the MCO may pay different rates, depending on the complexity of the individual case. These types of reimbursement systems are often quite difficult to administer, requiring both the MCO and the provider to keep records manually.

When there are a limited number of providers offering the ancillary service, it is more difficult to obtain substantial discounts and savings. Other than some types of exotic testing and therapy, this is usually not the case unless the MCO is located in a rural area. In general, good contracting makes it possible to achieve very high savings.

Contracting and Reimbursement for Pharmacy Services

Because they comprise such a high percentage of the total cost of health care, pharmacy services are especially important to managed care. The rate of inflation for pharmacy benefits has been higher in general than for any other single component of the health care dollar. This rapid and ongoing inflation in the cost of drug benefits is the result of increases in both the cost of drugs and in the total amount of drugs prescribed (Figure 3–6).

The advent of new and more effective drugs has led to an increase in the use of drug therapy. New drugs are available to replace problematic older drugs in the treatment of such conditions as high cholesterol and high blood pressure—conditions that lead to "silent diseases," so-called because they have

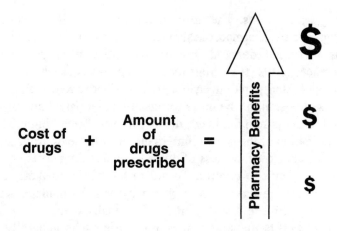

Figure 3-6 Factors causing pharmacy benefit cost inflation.

no obvious symptoms until the damage is severe (e.g., heart attack or stroke). Although the conditions had no symptoms, the drug treatments sometimes had side effects (e.g., niacin, administered for high cholesterol, causes flushing and heat flashes). Thus, many patients chose not to take any medication at all. With new, side effect–free drugs, treatment is widespread.

In other instances, new drugs have been created where there was no alternative at all, such as the current "viral cocktail" regimens for the treatment of acquired immunodeficiency syndrome (AIDS). New developments in existing classes of drugs, such as antidepressants, have increased usage, as physicians and patients search for the most effective drug in each case. Direct-to-consumer advertising by drug manufacturers has heightened the demand for certain drugs, such as new allergy medications. The introduction of so-called "lifestyle" drugs, such as pharmaceutical treatments for sexual dysfunction, has increased demand. Lastly, the creation of so-called "cosmeceuticals" (i.e., drugs for cosmetic effects), such as those for hair loss or skin rejuvenation, has also increased demand.

As almost all of the newer drugs are under patent and their production is monopolized, they tend to be priced high. The combination of the steep climb in the overall use of drugs and the current expensiveness of drugs has made drug costs especially difficult to control. To aid in the battle, virtually all MCOs use the services of a pharmacy benefits management company. In a few cases, the MCO actually owns the pharmacy benefits management company, but it is generally a free-standing company. As the name suggests, such a company specializes in managing drug benefits. The pharmacy benefits management company processes the claims for drugs submitted by the participating pharmacies, manages the formulary (i.e., the list of approved or recommended drugs), and monitors utilization. The MCO and pharmacy benefits management company work together to contract for a network of pharmacies, including a mail-order pharmacy, to provide the drug benefits for the MCO members. It is common for the pharmacy benefits management company to contract with national drugstore chains, as only the largest companies can usually provide the favorable pricing required under its contract with the MCO. Because the pharmacy benefits management company contracts with multiple chains, geographic coverage is usually very good, and even merely good geographic coverage is considered acceptable in return for the cost controls available through preferential pricing.

There are a few nontraditional methods of pharmacy reimbursement, such as capitation, but in general these have not been successful. The forces that have led to increasing drug costs have made it very difficult to predict and manage the risk for drug costs. Therefore, most pharmacies will not accept such risk, and pharmacy benefits management companies are reluctant to do so either.

The usual method of reimbursing pharmacies combines a fill-fee and the ingredient cost. The fill-fee is an amount that the pharmacy benefits management company pays the pharmacy simply for filling a prescription regardless of the drug prescribed. For example, a pharmacy benefits management company may pay a pharmacy two dollars for each prescription filled. The ingredient cost is the cost of the drug itself. It is not easy to determine the ingredient cost, because the price that a pharmacy pays a drug manufacturer may not be the same as another pharmacy. For example, nationwide chains are able to obtain lower prices (through their wholesale distributors) than small community pharmacies can obtain. It is common for the pharmacy benefits management company to refer to a standardized listing of drug prices and to reimburse based on that standard, often referred to as the average wholesale price. The pharmacy benefits management company commonly reimburses based on a percentage of the average wholesale price (e.g., 95 percent).

Pharmacy benefits management companies and MCOs (at least large ones) frequently negotiate a rebate from drug manufacturers. This approach does not apply to every drug, of course, but only to drugs that are relatively common and for which multiple good alternative therapies exist. For example, if there are 15 different nonsteroidal anti-inflammatory drugs (NSAIDs), the pharmacy benefits management company and the MCO may negotiate with the manufacturers of one or two of them to obtain rebates based on the inclusion of those drugs in the MCO's formulary. Inclusion in the formulary in this case represents preferential pricing, and the formulary will provide some type of indication that preferential pricing is in effect.

Contracting and Reimbursement for Behavioral Health Services

It is very common for MCOs to carve mental health and substance abuse services out when contracting for a medical care network. Because the management of behavioral health services is substantially different from the management of any other types of medical care, MCO medical managers turn to specialty organizations. (These services are often referred to as mental health and substance abuse [MH/SA] services but will be referred to here as behavioral health services.)

Generally, an MCO contracts with a specialty company in the behavioral health arena to build the behavioral health services network, reimburse the providers, and manage the cost and quality of the services provided. This organization may be a company or it may be a behavioral health specialty group or facility. If the MCO is an HMO or HMO-like, it might pay for behavioral health services through capitation. In other words, it might pay a specified amount per member to the behavioral health services organization, which then assumes full management of behavioral health services. The organization does not necessarily pay the actual service professionals through capitation, however. Like the arrangements with IPAs discussed earlier, the behavioral health services organization accepts financial risk but may pay the professionals on a different basis, such as fee-for-service or salary.

It is common for the network of behavioral health service providers to include substantially fewer than the total universe of available providers. In the case of behavioral health services, the size and scope of the network is particularly complex, as there are so many different types of service providers: psychiatrists, psychologists, therapists with a master's degree (e.g., master of social work [MSW]), therapists without a master's degree (e.g., licensed clinical social worker [LCSW]), and various types of substance abuse therapists. The behavioral health services organization usually determines the number and types of therapists that the network needs in order to provide adequate access and then contracts accordingly. Reimbursement of professionals, therefore, is usually on a fee-for-service basis, though capitation sometimes does occur when a large professional group takes on responsibility for all behavioral health services.

NETWORK MAINTENANCE AND MANAGEMENT

It is not enough to build a network. As noted earlier, there are many ongoing activities required of an MCO in order to maintain and manage the network. Recredentialing is an example of a common and required network maintenance activity. Related to this is the measurement and management of the performance of the network.

Among broad, network-based issues, access is primary. The MCO must ensure that the network is large enough and covers the proper geographic area to allow the MCO membership good access to all health care services. This means monitoring the number and types of provider practices by geographic location (usually ZIP code) and the number of practices actually open to members of the MCO in each location. For example, the MCO may be experiencing a high level of growth in a particular section of its service area, and the network management may need to recruit new providers in that area. Or the MCO may appear to have sufficient numbers of providers in an area, but many of those practices may be closed to new members (i.e., the providers are not accepting new patients). In this case, the MCO network management must recruit new providers as well as work with existing providers to see if they can or will open up their practices to new patients.

Individual providers, especially physicians, benefit from individual attention. The drug companies know this well, which is why they send sales representatives to visit physicians on an individual basis. Similarly, many MCOs require their network management departments to visit each provider at least once or twice a year. More attention may be paid in the case of providers who have specific issues. For example, some providers will have complex billing issues, or problems accessing member eligibility information; in such cases, additional time spent by network management staff may prevent further problems. Orientation of new providers and reorientation of existing providers to the way that the MCO operates are also individual-based activities.

On the less pleasant side, the MCO must occasionally deal with providers who are performing poorly, either financially or clinically (e.g., by providing substandard medical care or inadequate access to services). In each case, the MCO must either help the provider improve in the relevant areas or take action to remove the provider from the network. The termination of a contract with a provider, as noted earlier, is not easy to carry out and is likely to involve complex legal and regulatory issues. Fortunately, such actions are only rarely necessary.

CONCLUSION

An MCO's network of providers is its vehicle for providing health care to its members at an affordable cost. The composition of the network is directly dependent on the type of benefits plans being administered and has a direct bearing on the MCO's ability to manage the cost and quality of the care provided. Contractual terms between the providers and the MCO are a hallmark of managed care, and many of the provisions of such contracts are regulated. The maintenance of a network requires just as much work as does the original creation of the network.

Reimbursement of providers is an integral part of the overall management of utilization and quality of clinical services, but all provider payment systems are tools, not ends in themselves. Like all tools, reimbursement systems are useful only in the context of the other tools being used. Managing quality and utilization effectively is essential for achieving positive results; reimbursement schemes alone will never be enough.

CHAPTER 4

Medical Utilization and Quality

LEARNING OBJECTIVES

- Understand the basic components of utilization management
- Understand the different approaches to managing wellness and prevention, basic medical services, ancillary services, chronic diseases, and case management
- Understand the nature of external review
- Understand the basic components of quality management

The term *managed care* derives from the practice of managing certain aspects of the delivery of medical services as a way of controlling their cost. This cost, to oversimplify, is the result of two variables, price and volume. Chapter 3 briefly describes the price part of the equation (i.e., the reimbursement that providers receive). This chapter describes the volume part (i.e., the utilization of medical services). The term *utilization management* (UM) refers to the practice of managing medical services utilization.

Managed care organizations (MCOs) typically attempt to manage the quality of medical services as well. For some types of MCOs, such as health maintenance organizations (HMOs), quality management (QM) is required by law or regulation. A strong QM program can also be demanded by large employers or by accreditation programs such as those described in Chapter 6. In any case, MCOs have a moral obligation to implement a robust QM program in order to ensure that the medical services they deliver are of good quality.

The privacy requirements of the Health Insurance Portability and Accountability Act (HIPAA; see Chapter 6) and various state privacy laws set restrictions on access to medical information for purposes of UM and QM. For instance, the members of an MCO must give consent to having their medical information reviewed and must understand why it is being reviewed. Although the consent process can be cumbersome, it serves to protect patient confidentiality. In the event a member refuses to allow the MCO's medical management function to access his or her medical information, the MCO may reduce the benefits paid for services (the difference in coverage would be laid out in the member's description of benefits).

PREVENTION AND WELLNESS

Dr. Paul Elwood coined the term *health maintenance organization* to highlight the idea that HMOs were dedicated to providing preventive services. Indeed, whereas such services were not covered by most health insurance policies prior to the spread of HMOs, they have since become the norm.

Preventive services, unsurprisingly, are aimed at preventing certain diseases. They include childhood immunizations, which make up the most common type of preventive care. Other customary preventive services include adult immunizations, Pap smears, mammography, and screening for high cholesterol, high blood pressure, diabetes, and other widespread diseases.

Wellness programs are directed at helping members to change their lifestyles and develop healthy habits. These programs include nutrition (including weight management), smoking cessation, and various "healthy lifestyle" programs. Not every MCO provides a full range of wellness programs, however. Most HMOs do offer a wide assortment, but many preferred provider organizations (PPOs) and point-of-service (POS) plans (described in Chapter 2) offer only a few, such as smoking cessation programs, or none at all.

BASIC UTILIZATION MANAGEMENT

Utilization management encompasses prospective, concurrent, and retrospective activities (Figure 4–1). Prospective activities are intended to influence utilization before the fact, concur-

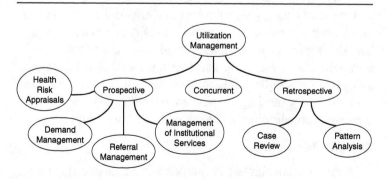

Figure 4–1 Components of utilization management.

rent activities are intended to influence utilization as it occurs, and retrospective activities include reviewing utilization patterns to determine where improvements need to be made.

Prospective Utilization Management

Prospective utilization management includes health risk appraisals, demand management, referral management, and management of institutional services.

Health Risk Appraisals

A health risk appraisal (HRA) is an overall assessment of a new patient's medical condition and risk factors. In managed care, HRAs are also designed to uncover information on member issues requiring intervention by the MCO to preserve health and lower overall costs. They may also be focused on specific lines of business or membership groups, such as commercial members, Medicare members, and Medicaid members.

Many advanced Medicare HMOs, in doing an HRA, go well beyond data-gathering forms and physical exams and actually send a nurse or home aid to the residence of a new member. During the visit, the nurse or aid may do a nutritional assessment, check for compliance with prescribed medications, and look for simple interventions that could save problems later, such as providing an inexpensive bath mat to prevent the member from slipping in the tub and breaking a hip.

Demand Management

Demand management is intended to influence the future demand for medical services. The most common demand management methods include providing

- access to preventive services
- convenient hours of operation
- medical advice manuals for use at home.

Recently, a more active method has shown considerable promise: providing a round-the-clock nurse advice line so that members, by calling a toll-free number, can access a trained nurse 24 hours a day, 7 days a week. The advice lines rely heavily on clinical protocols. Many MCOs that have advice lines have seen a decline in the use of their emergency departments.

Referral Management

Referral management is principally confined to HMOs, particularly HMOs that use the so-called gatekeeper model. In this model, a member's primary care provider (PCP) determines which medical services are truly necessary, coordinates the provision of these services, and protects against overuse of services. The provision of care by any health care professional other than the PCP must be authorized by the PCP. (Note that virtually all MCOs also offer coverage allowing women to have direct access to obstetricians and gynecologists.)

The authorization requirement allows the PCP to determine if a health problem or condition requires treatment by a specialist. If it does, the PCP authorizes a referral to a specialist under contract to the MCO. The authorization is seldom open-ended. It is usually for a limited number of visits (e.g., one to three) except in defined circumstances (e.g., chemotherapy is fully authorized for the entire course of treatment).

It is exceedingly rare for the MCO to become involved in the authorization process other than to capture the authorization data in order to process the claim properly. The PCP is expected to exercise proper clinical judgment without the MCO's intervention. The MCO should provide the PCP with periodic reports containing data on referral rates and costs as well as reports on the PCP's capitation pool or withhold if that is appropriate (see Chapter 3 for a discussion of capitation).

Management of Institutional Services

Prospective management of institutional services, both inpatient and outpatient, is a staple of managed care in all types of MCOs. The process is simple: someone calls the MCO to request authorization for an elective admission or outpatient procedure, the MCO checks the request against clinical criteria, and the MCO authorizes the procedure or not. In the case of an inpatient admission, the MCO usually assigns an expected length of stay as well.

Clinical criteria for authorization are commercially available, but the MCO may have developed its own criteria. Likewise, maximum allowable length of stay guidelines are commercially available, but the MCO may modify those guidelines to suit the local area. Most MCOs are now using computerized programs to determine quickly whether the clinical criteria are met and to capture pertinent data.

Who calls the MCO for authorization depends on the type of health benefits plan. For indemnity insurance plans or for the out-of-network benefits in PPOs and POS plans, the member must call or face an economic penalty. For HMOs and the in-network benefits in PPOs and POS plans, the burden of responsibility is on the provider, and it is the provider who suffers an economic penalty for failure to comply.

The economic penalties vary based on the type of health benefits plan. If authorization is obtained before the admission or procedure takes place, there is no penalty. If authorization is not obtained, a penalty will be imposed. In some cases, the penalty is noncoverage (e.g., this would be the penalty in an HMO with no out-of-plan benefits). In a PPO or a POS plan, the penalty may be a higher level of coinsurance (e.g., 50 percent of the cost of the service). In an emergency situation, a penalty is not imposed as long as the MCO is notified within a reasonable period of time (usually one business day after the admission).

Concurrent Utilization Management

Concurrent review of utilization, also known as continued stay review, applies almost exclusively to inpatient care and to complex, expensive cases. An MCO, such as an indemnity or service plan, a PPO, or a large HMO with numerous network hospitals, will typically perform a concurrent review from a remote site via telephone. The MCO's UM nurse will call the hospital to ascertain the status of the case. If the case is on track, no further action is taken. If the hospital stay is going to exceed the previously authorized days, the UM nurse will collect clinical data and either authorize the additional days or deny coverage for them. Rather than deny coverage, however, the UM nurse is far more likely to work with the physician and the hospital's own utilization review and discharge planning department to facilitate the patient's discharge. For example, home physical therapy or outpatient treatments may be arranged.

Many HMOs will send a UM nurse to the hospital in order to obtain more detailed and timely information and more actively manage the case. The process is otherwise the same as described above, but communications and information exchange are better than when only the telephone is used.

In the event of ambiguity or disagreement during the concurrent review process, the UM nurse refers the case to a physician working with or for the MCO (either the medical director or a physician advisor). This physician may call the attending physician to discuss the case and may then make a determination regarding authorization for further payments. If the attending physician and the medical director cannot agree on the need for or the appropriateness of the care, an external review process may be used, as described later in this chapter.

Retrospective Utilization Management

Retrospective utilization management activities fall into two broad categories, case review and pattern analysis.

Case Review

In case review, past cases are examined for appropriateness of care, billing errors, or other problems. If an error or irregularity is found in a particular case, the MCO may adjust payment or at least investigate the case. If there is some suspicion that a provider is chronically making errors or even committing fraud, the MCO may place the provider on regular review.

In almost all instances, the case review process is routine, and any problems discovered are the result of simple errors by providers. The vast majority of providers would never engage in fraud, but there is always the possibility that one or a few will, and the MCO must be on the alert for cheating. If fraud is detected, the MCO must determine whether the case is serious enough to warrant notifying the authorities or instead try to deal with the provider by itself—by demanding that the money be returned, for example, and then removing the provider from the network. In more serious cases and in cases involving Medicare, the MCO must notify law enforcement agencies.

Pattern Analysis

Pattern analysis involves the amassing of significant amounts of utilization data to determine if patterns exist. These patterns may be provider specific (e.g., over- or underutilization of certain tests or procedures) or planwide (e.g., an unanticipated increase in cardiac testing costs). After a pattern has been found, the reasons for it must be investigated so that corrective action may be taken.

MCOs are now attempting to provide more extensive retrospective data to the network providers to allow the providers to compare themselves to their peers and modify their own practices as appropriate. This form of feedback promises to be a powerful additional tool for controlling health care costs and quality.

EXTERNAL REVIEW PROGRAMS

Most MCOs are required to provide for external review of disputed coverage decisions. In the review process, outside specialists (i.e., specialty physicians who do not work for the MCO) look at the relevant facts of a particular decision to determine whether the MCO should provide coverage for medical services for which it has denied coverage. External reviews are not common, and when they occur, they typically involve treatments that are experimental or would generally be considered medically unnecessary.

Here's how the review process might come into play. Suppose that a member of an MCO has a continuing severe medical condition and that the attending physician recommends a risky or experimental procedure, such as a transplant. Given the likely assumption that the MCO's benefits policy excludes coverage for experimental or unproven procedures, the MCO may decide this procedure falls into the unproven category and deny coverage. The attending physician, however, might dispute that the procedure is actually experimental and argue instead that it should be covered. If the medical director of the MCO remains unbending, the member (through the physician, usually) could then request an external review. The MCO then would contact a panel of specialists who are in the same specialty as the attending physician but do not work for the MCO (other than doing external reviews), and, with the consent of the member, it would provide these external reviewers with relevant medical information. The member and the attending physician would also provide whatever information they wish to the panel. The panel may hold a hearing or discuss the case with the attending physician and the medical director, but whatever the process, it will eventually issue a determination as to whether the MCO is liable for coverage of the procedure. That decision is then binding upon the MCO.

External review programs are required in many states. Federal legislation requiring external review programs has been debated as well. However, at this time no federal legisation has been passed. Although one might think that appeals would generally be granted, the truth is that the denial of coverage is upheld about as often as it is overturned.

DISEASE AND CASE MANAGEMENT

Disease management and case management focus on conditions that are chronic, expensive to treat, or both (Table 4–1). It is no surprise to anyone that a small percentage of members of an MCO account for a very large percentage of the MCO's total medical costs. Although the majority of members have routine medical needs, some have serious chronic medical conditions—such as severe diabetes, acquired immunodeficiency syndrome (AIDS), or certain heart conditions—that require a great deal of expensive medical care. Likewise, certain acute cases—such as a severe automobile accident or a very premature newborn—are also expensive.

The related functions of large-case management and disease management are designed to address the medical needs of members requiring very expensive care. By paying particular attention to these members, the MCO is able to lower costs while improving outcomes and quality.

Case Management

Case management of catastrophic or chronic cases, whose costs often exceed routine costs by several orders of magnitude, has the potential to deliver substantial savings. In this type of utilization management, trained nurses coordinate aspects of care, such as rehabilitation, home care, health education, and the like, and thereby improve outcomes as well as reduce expenses.

Table 4–1 Comparison of Conventional Case Management and Disease Management

	Case Management	Disease Management
Goal	Reduce per case cost, improve episodic care	Reduce per disease cost, improve patient outcomes
Emphasis	Appropriate treatment of illness, use of alternative settings	Improved management of chronic care, prevention and education for patients, families, and physicians
Scope	Patient often has multiple diseases	Patient is initially evaluated for a single disease
Review	Periodic concurrent review	Prospective and concurrent review
Guidelines	Generic, externally imposed	Customized to diagnosis, internally designed
Caregivers	Generalists, nurses	Specialists, multidisciplinary team
Data sources	Primarily inpatient (tracks length of stay, profit margin per confinement, mortality)	All points of service (tracks annual episode of care cost, medication compliance, functional status)
Integration	Isolated medical management	Integrated medical management
Risk	Lacks ability to bear financial risk	Increased ability to bear financial risk

Source: Adapted from D.W. Plocher, Disease Management, in *The Managed Health Care Handbook,* 3rd ed., p. 321, © 1996, Aspen Publishers, Inc.

Disease Management

Disease management is a special form of case management in which the MCO focuses on a handful of selected diseases and works proactively with each patient to control the disease's course. The usual result is greater continuity and a better outcome. Much attention is directed toward trying to make the patient's condition better through different approaches or at least preventing it from getting worse. The hallmark of a disease management program is the inclusion of numerous types of health professionals, not just physicians. For example, a clinical pharmacist may play a more active role in treating childhood asthma than the pediatrician (e.g., by teaching the child how to use inhaled steroids). Likewise, a dietitian may be of great service to patients with a severe heart condition by teaching them how to maintain a good diet and avoid unhealthy habits.

ANCILLARY AND PHARMACEUTICAL SERVICES

Ancillary Services

Ancillary services, described in Chapter 3, are medical services that are not personally provided by physicians and are not hospital or institutional services. The two common types are diagnostic services and therapeutic services. As noted in Chapter 3, ancillary diagnostic services include laboratory, radiology, nuclear testing, computed tomography (CT), magnetic resonance imaging (MRI), electroencephalography, and cardiac testing. Ancillary therapeutic services include cardiac rehabilitation, noncardiac rehabilitation, physical therapy, occupational therapy, and speech therapy.

The management of ancillary diagnostic and therapeutic services makes use of several approaches (Figure 4–2). First, excessive ordering of ancillary services by some physicians can often be reduced through practice profiling and feedback as well as direct discussions between the medical director and these physicians.

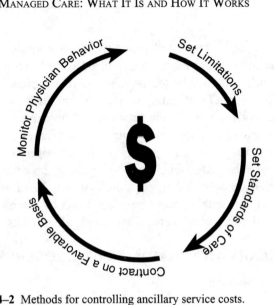

Figure 4–2 Methods for controlling ancillary service costs.

Another strategy is to limit the number and duration of certain types of ancillary services that can be authorized at once, at least on a routine basis. For example, an MCO may allow only three weeks of routine physical therapy services to be authorized initially; if additional weeks of therapy are needed, they would require an additional authorization. The restriction on the original authorization forces the physician to reassess the case and determine whether the services are still useful.

For a small number of expensive services not commonly used, the MCO may put into place standards of care. Before ordering an expensive test, for example, a physician might have to suspect a particular diagnosis (one that the test pertains to) rather than prescribe the test just to see what turns up.

One important way of controlling the cost of ancillary services is through favorable contracting. Although favorable contracting has already been discussed (in Chapter 3), it is such a cornerstone of cost control that it bears mentioning here. Capitation is well suited to ancillary services in HMOs and some POS plans, but favorable contracting can deliver substantial savings for any type of MCO. The basic principle is to develop ancillary service provider–MCO contracts according to which the providers charge the MCO reduced fees in return for being part of a restricted network and getting referrals from the MCO. The contracts should include quality and service requirements that providers must meet and should offer the providers financial incentives for meeting these requirements.

Pharmaceutical Services

Drug benefits are unique. The cost of drugs accounts for a large part of the health care dollar—between 10 and 17 percent of total health care costs for the typical MCO. Until managed care became prevalent, prescription drugs, like preventive care services, were not even covered by insurance. Now it is rare for an MCO not to provide coverage for drugs, although the benefits differ from plan to plan.

Not only do drug costs constitute a major portion of health care spending, the rate of inflation for drugs has been much higher than for any other area of health care. One reason is that individual drugs are increasingly expensive; another is that far more drugs are being prescribed than ever before. Many new drugs have been developed in the past 10 years, and physicians can now treat certain conditions far more effectively with these drugs than previously. But the growing use of pharmacotherapy comes at a price, since new drugs are generally expensive.

Most MCOs contract with an outside organization to manage their pharmacy benefits (Exhibit 4–1). Organizations of this type are commonly called *pharmacy benefits management companies (PBMs)*. PBMs rarely assume financial risk for drug costs but are responsible for all aspects of management. A PBM will typically contract with many MCOs to grow large enough to achieve economies of scale as well as negotiate better financial terms (see Chapter 3).

In managing drug benefits for an MCO, a PBM makes use of the following elements, among other less important ones.

Formulary

A formulary is a list of drugs covering typical medical needs, although it does not include all of the available drugs

---

Exhibit 4–1 Why Managed Care Organizations Contract with Pharmacy Benefits Management Companies

Formulary. A PBM may negotiate discounted rates with manufacturers of certain drugs listed in the formulary.

Drug utilization review (DUR). Contract allows PBM or MCO to manage volume and nature of prescriptions as well as provide special authorization for certain drugs.

Benefits design. Contract provides for lower costs when members resort to less expensive alternatives.

for each medical condition. In many cases, several drugs are equally useful for a particular condition but differ widely in price. In addition, the PBM, because of its size, may have negotiated volume discounts with the manufactures of certain of those drugs. The formulary, then, contains drugs that are effective and are the least costly among the alternatives. If one particular drug is clearly the most effective, that drug will be the one listed on the formulary regardless of cost.

The PBM provides the MCO with a formulary, which is then modified by the MCO's pharmacy and therapeutics (P&T) committee to meet the needs of the network physicians. For example, the P&T committee may determine that a drug not on the formulary really needs to be included and will ensure that it is. More often, the P&T committee reviews requests for exceptions. A physician or member might desire to use a drug not on the formulary, and the P&T committee would consider the pros and cons of allowing use of the drug. Requests for exceptions almost always involve highly expensive and infrequently used drugs (such as growth hormone) for which the indications for use are not always clear.

Drug Utilization Review

Drug utilization review (DUR) consists of activities and strategies for managing the volume and pattern of prescriptions. The most common DUR strategy is to create prescribing profiles and provide the profile information to the physicians so that they can compare their prescribing patterns to those of their peers.

Another common strategy is to require special authorization for certain drugs. Authorization requirements are usually restricted to a very small list of drugs that have the potential for being prescribed inappropriately. The example of growth hormone was mentioned above. An MCO would want to be sure that growth hormone was being prescribed for children who are truly suffering a deficiency rather than for children who are smaller than average or have parents who want their children to be bigger.

Benefits Design

Though not technically a utilization management function, the design of prescription drug benefits is an important element of the overall approach. One simple strategy for affecting utilization is to charge members a lower co-payment for using less expensive alternatives. For example, if the prescription is filled with a generic equivalent, the co-payment might be $5; if it is filled with a brand-name drug, the co-pay would rise to $10.

Recently, the use of three co-payment tiers has become widespread. In this type of benefits design, the lowest co-payment (e.g., $5) is for generic drugs, the middle amount (e.g., $10) is for brand-name drugs that are on the formulary, and the highest amount (e.g., $25) is for brand-name drugs that are not on the formulary but that the member wants to have nonetheless. In all cases, the pharmacies under contract to the PBM are supposed to provide information to members about alternatives to the most expensive drugs.

QUALITY MANAGEMENT

MCOs vary in their approach to medical quality management. Indemnity and service plans and even PPOs generally are somewhat less aggressive in managing quality than are HMOs, although, like all generalizations, there are notable exceptions. As in utilization management, as model types progress through the continuum, greater attention is paid to managing quality and more resources are expended on this task. Almost all MCOs begin the quality management process by verifying the credentials of participating providers (see Chapter 3).

Beyond credential verification, MCOs generally employ two approaches to quality management, often together: classic quality management and total quality management (or continuous quality improvement). Following is a brief description of these approaches.

Classic Quality Management

The classic approach to managing quality is based on the works of Avedis Donabedian. The three key elements are structure, process, and outcome (Figure 4–3).

Structure

The task here is to look at how the infrastructure of the MCO is related to quality and to make changes in the infrastructure to bring about quality improvements. Structure studies might, for instance, examine medical records (e.g., to verify the presence of a drug allergies list or review laboratory notes), immunization records, access to care (e.g., the length of time between calling to make a routine or urgent appointment and the appointment date), waiting times in the office, telephone responsiveness, and so forth. These studies are usu-

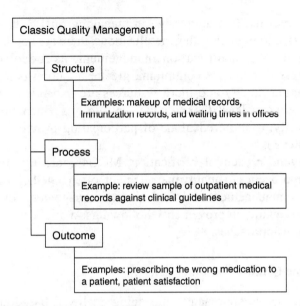

Figure 4–3 Classic quality management.

ally done on-site by the MCO's quality management nurses. A special type of structure study examines the effect of the utilization system on access to care. In particular, the MCO gathers data to discover whether utilization is inappropriately low and whether the authorization system is acting as a barrier to necessary care.

Process

The care process is the way in which care is actually rendered. To investigate the care process, MCO nurses typically review a sample of outpatient medical records in light of the clinical guidelines established by the quality management committee. Clinical guidelines are specific to a particular disease or procedure. For example, guidelines on the diagnosis and treatment of ear infections are common and typically include the steps of the history and physical exam that a physician should record and the appropriate types of treatment and follow-up that should occur. Guidelines are also common for inpatient care, such as for the diagnosis and treatment of heart attacks (early detection and aggressive treatment of heart attacks have been shown to be beneficial, as has the use of beta-blockers after discharge).

After reviewing the medical records and measuring compliance, the nurses report back to the providers and the MCO. The MCO notes deficiencies and clearly states what corrective actions need to be taken. For example, despite the known usefulness of beta-blockers, many patients who have had heart attacks are discharged from the hospital without being placed on these drugs. The MCO will provide feedback to physicians who are not prescribing beta-blockers and indicate that their prescription is the standard of practice (unless there is a good medical reason countering their use, such as the presence of congestive heart failure). After a suitable period of time has passed, the MCO will conduct an identical study to ensure that appropriate changes in practice behavior have occurred.

Outcome

In evaluating the outcome of care, MCOs generally look at adverse events and MCO-wide measures. Adverse events are negative outcomes that could have been prevented, such as a hospital-acquired infection. Medical errors, such as prescribing or dispensing the wrong drug, make up a special category and have recently been recognized as more common than previously imagined. An MCO will conduct studies to look for medical errors and report the data back to the providers, along with guidelines to help prevent errors. It must be noted that providers themselves, especially hospital systems, are well aware of the pervasiveness of medical errors and are working independently to prevent them.

An MCO will perform outcomes studies to uncover whether its providers are generally successful at treating designated conditions. It might, for example, look at the rate for control of hypertension without preventable side effects, the rate for delivery of healthy babies, and so forth. The MCO will choose conditions that occur often enough to measure and then determine what represents a good outcome. Defining a good outcome is not as easy as it seems, since many conditions cannot be cured, only controlled. The quality management committee is responsible for choosing what types of outcomes to measure and how to determine if an outcome is successful or not.

If the rate of successful outcomes for a given condition is not acceptable, the MCO quality management function may study that condition further, using structure and process studies as well. An example will serve to illustrate how these studies can work together. Suppose the MCO chooses to look at the outcomes of cardiac bypass surgery. The study discovers high success rates except at one hospital. The MCO analyzes the data and finds that patients who have surgery at that hospital end up going back to surgery (i.e., being operated on a second time) much more often than do patients who have surgery at other hospitals. The MCO then conducts a process study, which uncovers the fact that the hospital's standards of care for postoperative care (i.e., care given immediately after surgery) do not contain the same infection control requirements found in other hospitals. At this point, there may be enough information for the hospital (and the physicians, of course) to change what they are doing to correct the problem. But to take the example one step further, suppose that a structure study shows that the machine used for sterilizing certain instruments is not being serviced properly. The incorrect servicing and the difference in infection control requirements together would be considered the likely root causes of the postoperative infections and the lower success rate for cardiac bypass surgery experienced by the one hospital.

Member satisfaction is among the outcomes an MCO might study. The MCO will typically survey members regularly, analyze complaints, and so forth, to determine overall satisfaction levels and to act on identified problems. As noted in Chapter 6, Medicare requires that special types of member satisfaction surveys be performed by any MCO that has Medicare+Choice members. Accreditation agencies also require member satisfaction surveys.

TOTAL QUALITY MANAGEMENT

Managed care has adopted many of the tenets of the approach to industrial quality improvement referred to as *total quality management (TQM)* or *continuous quality improvement (CQI)*. This approach makes most sense for closed-panel

MCOs, but all types of MCOs can benefit from TQM techniques. Although these techniques can be quite complex, the basic strategy is simple—to continually reexamine what is done and how it is done with the goal of doing it better. In other words, the strategy is to not stop with good enough but to strive continually to do better.

Whereas the classical approach to quality management focuses on conforming to standards, TQM emphasizes the importance of improving the standards. These two approaches are not inconsistent. The only way to know if the medical care provided by an MCO conforms to the current best practices is to document these practices and measure the care provided against them. But practices change, and the goal of TQM is search out new best practices and ensure medical care changes to conform to these.

The medical practices MCOs address tend to be different than the ones that health researchers address. For instance, health researchers at a teaching hospital may perform rigorous clinical studies to determine which of two clinical protocols (i.e., ways to deliver care) is better. These studies are commonly used to evaluate treatments for cancer, AIDS, and so forth. MCOs may participate in such studies but are rarely their primary sponsors. Instead, MCOs focus their quality improvement efforts on issues directly under their control. Common examples include finding better ways to notify members about needed preventive care (e.g., immunizations and mammograms), better ways to identify drug interactions, and better ways to help patients recover faster following surgery.

CONCLUSION

There are a handful of factors that distinguish managed care from indemnity health insurance. The presence, in managed care, of a contracted network of providers and favorable pricing is one such differentiator. However, simply obtaining a better price for medical services, while necessary for controlling costs, is not by itself any indication that health care is being managed. It is the management of utilization and quality that truly sets managed care apart.

Utilization management and quality management are constantly evolving. What worked well 10 to 15 years ago is now less valuable and in some cases has even been abandoned. As MCOs and providers become more sophisticated in dealing with issues of overutilization and variable quality of care, managed care will change to take advantage of the improvements.

CHAPTER 5

Internal Operations

LEARNING OBJECTIVES

- Understand the basic components of the internal operations of managed care organizations
- Understand the differences between marketing and sales
- Understand the basic concepts of underwriting, premium billing, and financial management
- Understand the application of medical policy and claims payment
- Understand the various components of member services

The vast majority of employees of any MCO are involved in activities that are administrative and not directly related to the provision of medical care. Further, whereas 83 to 95 percent of the total health care dollar is spent on clinical services, most MCOs seek to control costs mainly in the administrative area. In fact, for any MCO member, most of the member's interactions with the MCO will essentially administrative in nature, whether the member is applying for an identification card or resolving a complex claim for medical services.

Many administrative services may be seen as "middle man" services and viewed as adding little value. Indeed, during the mid-1990s, *middle man* was used as a pejorative term, and providers and consumers alike tended to believe that administrative services were largely a waste of money. Consequently, many providers attempted to take over administrative functions themselves to "cut out the middle man." As noted earlier, almost all of these attempts ended in disaster. Whatever the attitude of providers toward these services, there is no question but that the services are complex, are specialized, and must be done. Furthermore, whether a particular type of service actually adds value is subjective (i.e., the answer depends on who is considering the issue). Does a regulation requiring the creation of yet another report add value? To regulators, the answer might be a clear yes; to an MCO, the answer will likely be less apparent.

MARKETING AND SALES

There can be no MCO if there are no enrolled members. Therefore, the first critical operational activities an MCO must undertake are to market its services and sell its products to target audiences. The terms *marketing* and *sales* are often used synonymously, although marketing is not quite the same as sales. Marketing involves creating a strategy for entering a market and building the infrastructure needed to sell the MCO's services. Sales, on the other hand, is the actual activity of selling to those in a position to buy.

By way of illustration, the marketing department may determine that the MCO should target large employers in its service area. It would then identify these employers, the issues that might make the MCO attractive to them, the best approach to selling the MCO's products to them, and so forth. The marketing department is also responsible for creating supporting material, such as brochures and descriptions of the MCO's offerings, as well as advertising, public relations, and other broad activities designed to increase the visibility and enhance the reputation of the MCO in the market.

The sales staff, on the other hand, are responsible for contacting the large employers and meeting with the benefits managers. Personal discussions with the benefits manager of an employer allows the MCO's sales representative to find out the employer's priorities when it comes to purchasing health care benefits for employees and to describe what the MCO offers that would be of value to the employer. The sales representative also discusses financial terms, guides the employer to through various benefits design options, and so forth. In other words, all of the activities that involve face-to-face dealing with customers are the domain of the sales staff. (Note that the premium rates that the MCO will charge customers are set by the underwriting department. It is this department that analyzes the likely medical costs for a given employer and determines what products to offer and what rates to charge for those products.)

Market Segmentation

The market for managed care is not uniform, and it is important to understand the differences between the various segments. First, the market may be thought of having wholesale and retail components. The wholesale component consists of employers, whereas the retail component consists of individual consumers. In most cases, an MCO will market and sell to both components.

Segmentation by organizational size is also common. Large employers purchase services far differently than do small employers, and mid-sized employers occupy, well, the middle ground. Therefore, it is common for the sales department of an MCO to organize its internal operations around segments based on organizational size. The sales department might also separately treat (1) national businesses with widely scattered locations, (2) local employers, and (3) individuals not covered through an employer (the individual purchaser market). Further market segmentation often exists, even within each broad category, but a more detailed discussion of the topic is not warranted here.

Wholesale versus Retail

The wholesale side of managed care involves the marketing and selling of managed care products to employers and government agencies, such as the state Medicaid program or the armed forces. The size of the employer or organization is irrelevant. The retail side of managed care involves the selling of products to individual employees without the intervention of an employer or organization (Figure 5–1).

The importance of the distinction between the wholesaling and retailing of managed care is that most mid-sized and large employers give their employees the option of choosing a health benefits plan from one of several MCOs, and even

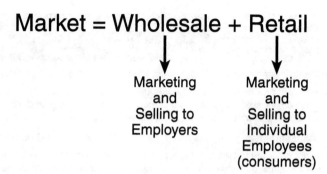

Market = Wholesale + Retail

Marketing and Selling to Employers

Marketing and Selling to Individual Employees (consumers)

Figure 5–1 Wholesale versus retail.

---

when one MCO is used exclusively, the MCO typically will offer several different plans (e.g., a high option plan and a low option plan). A commercial sale begins with a sale to a group (the wholesale), and it is this sale that allows the MCO's products and services to be offered to employees in the first place.

Large Employer Groups

Large employers, roughly defined as employers having more than 3,000 employees, are usually self-insured (Figure 5–2. Note: there is little agreement about when to start calling an employer a "large employer," and many in the industry would use 2,000 or even 1,000 employees to identify and employer as "large"). Self-insured employers bear the financial risk for medical expenses themselves rather than purchasing insurance to protect against the financial risk. As noted elsewhere in this book, assuming the financial risk for medical

Small Employer Groups	Mid-Sized Employer Groups	Large Employer Groups

Small employer groups (subsegments: 10 lives and less; 10–50 lives).

This segment represents the largest number of employer firms. These are true small businesses. This segment is regulatory driven and plan design tends to be simple with funding on a guaranteed cost basis.

Mid-sized employer groups (subsegments: 50–250 lives; 250–3,000 lives).

This represents the middle market where employers at the lower end tend to behave like small business. As the employee size increases, so does the employer's need for sophisticated services that are managed by a dedicated company individual who is responsible for the design and management of the benefit program. Multisite dimension appears. Benefit funding moves toward risk retention by the employer.

Large employer groups (more than 3,000 lives).

The large employer generally has many sites and diversity of needs. Choice of plan for large and national employers is typically experience rating or self-funding as the predominant funding design.

Figure 5–2 Market size segmentation and characteristics. *Source:* Reprinted from G. Marcus and J.C. Thomson, Sales and Marketing in Managed Health Care Plans: The Process of Distribution, in *The Managed Health Care Handbook,* 4th ed., P.R. Kongstvedt, ed., p. 805, © 2000, Aspen Publishers, Inc.

---

expenses allows them to avoid paying state insurance premium taxes and also to avoid state-imposed requirements, such as mandated benefits, mandated inclusion of certain providers, and state-specific appeals and grievance programs. Furthermore, large employers often have sites in different geographic areas or even in different states.

Large employers purchase health benefits for their employees primarily through specialized health benefits consulting firms. This type of firm charges fees to the employer for its services and receives no income from the MCO as part of each sale.

Since a self-insured employer is taking on the financial risk for medical expenses itself, it is primarily interested in an MCO's ability to administer the benefits program it wishes to provide its employees. A benefits consulting firm helps to design the actual benefits package and then determines the requirements that an MCO must meet to administer this package. Large employers commonly require any MCO they contract with to

- provide adequate network access to care (defined by the number of available providers per geographic area)
- act in a timely fashion in paying claims, resolving problems or complaints, and so forth
- be certified by a recognized accreditation agency (see Chapter 7)
- offer medical management performance guarantees

The cost of administrative services is subject to intense negotiation, with the employer wishing to pay as little as possible while demanding a high level of performance. Self-insured employers also typically purchase stop-loss insurance (or reinsurance) to protect against the cost of catastrophic cases.

Despite the number of large employers that are self-insured, when an individual who has health benefits coverage from a large company sees a provider, the provider (and the member of the MCO, for that matter) typically assumes that, since the member is carrying an identification card with the MCO's name on it, the MCO is providing the insurance. Obviously, the provider could easily be mistaken. Instead, it might be the employer that is providing the insurance, determining the benefits package, and so forth, in which case the MCO would simply be administering the benefits plan on behalf of the employer.

Small Employer Groups

Small employers, roughly defined as having between 2 and 50 employees, occupy the opposite end of the spectrum. These employers are unable to afford the risk of self-insuring and therefore do purchase group health benefits insurance from an MCO. A small employer usually has a single site or several sites in a restricted geographic area (exceptions occur, of course). It is unusual for a small employer to offer more than one type of health benefits plan or contract with more than one MCO because of underwriting risks associated with having more than one insurance carrier in a small account.

In the case of a small employer, the wholesale is really the entire sale, since the employees do not have multiple carriers to choose from. (Of course, many employees have working spouses with access to health benefits plans, and these employees can choose to forgo coverage and depend on the coverage of their spouses.)

A small employer may purchase health benefits coverage directly from an MCO but usually a broker facilitates the sale. The broker helps the small employer find appropriate health benefits coverage, provides advice, and usually receives as ongoing revenue a percentage of the premium payment that the employer makes to the MCO.

Mid-sized Employer Groups

The dividing lines between small, medium, and large employers are of course arbitrary. At the extreme ends—that is, in the case of very small and very large employers—the ways an MCO markets and sells services are definable. In the middle things are muddier, although the larger an employer is, the greater the likelihood it will use a consultant rather than a broker (Figure 5–3) and will self-insure rather than purchase insurance. The transition to use of a consultant and to self-insuring occurs at no set point, but it frequently happens when an employer grows to be around 500 employees.

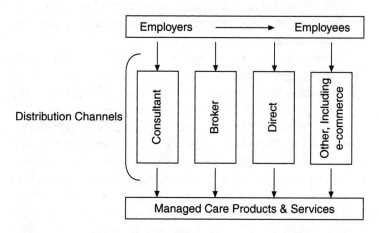

Figure 5–3 Distribution channels. *Source:* Reprinted from G. Marcus and J.C. Thomson, Sales and Marketing in Managed Health Care Plans: The Process of Distribution in *The Managed Health Care Handbook,* 4th ed., P.R. Kongstvedt, ed., p. 806, © 2000, Aspen Publishers, Inc.

Individual Purchasers

Individuals purchase health insurance or managed care in fundamentally different ways than do groups. Medicare beneficiaries are individual purchasers of a sort, but the dynamics of the Medicare market are so unusual as to warrant separate discussion of this market (see Chapter 6).

Individuals have much greater difficulty buying health insurance of any kind than do employee groups, for example. Their ability to acquire health insurance is affected by state laws and regulations and by the Health Insurance Portability and Accountability Act of 1996 (see Chapter 7), and in general it is directly related to their age, sex, and existing medical conditions. This does not mean that an individual who is older or has an existing medical condition cannot purchase health insurance, although there are circumstances in which this is so.

Individuals who are younger and have no medical conditions that require ongoing care usually are able to purchase health insurance policies at reasonable rates. The policies may exclude certain conditions, however. For example, individual policies commonly exclude pregnancy because of the risk that a woman will buy an insurance policy covering pregnancy services, get pregnant, make use of the covered services, then drop the policy, preventing the insurance company or MCO from ever recovering the cost of the health care provided. Some states do not allow such exclusions, and in those states the price of all individual policies must be raised substantially in order to pay for the services of those who use them and cancel their policies soon thereafter.

Not all MCOs or insurance companies offer individual policies. Those that do may be required to do so under state laws that mandate a so-called open enrollment period—a period in which each MCO must accept any person who applies for coverage. In a state where a mandated open enrollment period exists, individual policies typically are expensive and are not marketed or sold except as required by state law (e.g., the state may require the MCOs to advertise during defined periods and via defined types of notices). MCOs that actively market to individuals usually do their marketing through brokers. An individual applying for coverage must pass underwriting criteria before a policy is issued (see the section on underwriting below).

There are many circumstances in which a person has the right to purchase an individual health insurance policy. For instance, if the person has recently lost coverage under a group policy (e.g., as a result of being laid off) or is able to prove continuous coverage by another carrier, he or she has the right to purchase coverage. This does not mean that the cost of the health policy will be low, however. Since the individual purchaser market is such that people can drop their health insurance policies whenever they want or not buy insurance in the first place (i.e., unlike in the case of auto insurance, no one is compelled by law to purchase health insurance), healthier and younger people tend not to buy individual health insurance policies, while older and less healthy people do. Therefore, the overall risk for medical costs tends to be higher than normal in most health plans in which people have a right to buy individual insurance policies.

Determining What To Sell

Every MCO offers multiple products, and the sales department must determine what products and services to sell to each employer. An employer may have a firm idea of what type of product it wants, but usually it will want to balance the various factors in making its purchasing decisions, and the sales staff will work with the employer to weigh these factors. The factors an employer will consider in choosing a health benefits plan include the cost of the plan, the degree of coverage provided, the degree of access to network care, and the size of the network (Figure 5–4).

The MCO will have an array of standard products in each broad category (e.g., HMO, POS plan, and PPO). For example, plans may require different levels of co-payment for office visits, offer different levels of drug coverage, and so forth. If the employer is a large one, it will, via its benefits consultants, typically create specialized benefits plans (e.g., plans that have special limitations on coverage for certain conditions). The sales staff, in conjunction with the underwriting staff, must work with the employer to determine the cost and feasibility of the options the employer wishes to consider.

ENROLLMENT AND BILLING

Enrollment and billing are straightforward MCO functions. The enrollment and billing department ensures that new mem-

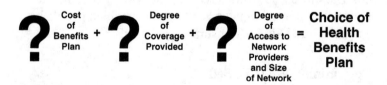

Figure 5–4 How to choose a health plan.

bers are entered into the MCO's information systems, identification cards are generated and issued, and so forth. Ongoing maintenance of membership files is also a critical function.

There are many circumstances where a member's eligibility for health benefits must be verified. For instance, a hospital will want to confirm that a patient is covered under a health plan in order to properly bill the MCO or health insurer. If it is not possible for the hospital to verify eligibility, it will make other payment arrangements with the patient. Another example concerns capitation. Capitation payments are actually prepayments for services. These payments should only be made for members who are actually covered by the MCO and whose premiums have been paid. If the MCO has not updated its membership database, it will incorrectly make capitation payments for former members and also will fail to pay providers proper capitation for recently joined members.

The MCO bills employers based on enrolled members. The seemingly simple activity of billing is actually quite complex and prone to error. In any company, employees are hired and employees leave throughout the year. Thus, the membership database must be updated each month. However, updating is not always practical, especially in an MCO with thousands of employer customers.

In addition, employers are not always good about notifying MCOs about employment changes. Further, as might be expected, terminations constitute a far worse problem than hirings. New employees want their health coverage to become effective immediately, and thus they have a reason to go through enrollment, but employers often have no formal process for disenrolling employees when they leave (voluntarily or not). Even employers that have a formal process do not always notify the MCO in a timely manner.

The drawbacks of carrying ineligible members as active members are obvious. First, the MCO may pay for health benefits services for individuals whose premium payments have not been received. Second, the MCO may pay capitation for such individuals. In addition, the MCO will believe that it is entitled to receive premium payments for such individuals and will book the revenue (though it has not received the cash) as accounts receivable. Correcting the mistake results in a negative revenue adjustment.

CLAIMS

The claims department is responsible for ensuring that the providers are paid for their services and that members who have paid providers out of pocket receive the reimbursement they are entitled to. The role of the claims department is consistently underappreciated by individuals who do not understand how an MCO operates.

To the naïve, paying claims seems like it should be entirely straightforward: a claim comes in, a check goes out. What could be complex about that? Plenty. In fact, the claims functions affect and are affected by all other areas within the MCO, as indicated in the following discussion.

Administration of Benefits

At the most basic level, the claims department administers the health coverage benefits of the MCO. In the case of capitation, the finance department usually pays the providers, although the claims department may still process encounters (i.e., claims submitted by capitated providers that are counted for purposes of data capture but are not paid). However, as pointed out in Chapter 3, in all but a few MCOs, those that globally capitate IDSs, the vast majority of health care services generate claims that must be paid.

The most common function performed by the claims department is to determine the extent of coverage (i.e., what health services are covered by the MCO) and under what circumstances a benefit does or does not apply. To illustrate this function, a simplified benefits administration scenario is given below.

Suppose an employer has purchased a POS benefits package that provides for a $10 co-pay with no deductible for visits to a primary care physician (PCP), a $15 co-pay with no deductible for specialist visits authorized by the PCP, and a 20-percent coinsurance requirement with a $200 deductible for services not authorized by the PCP.

When a claim from a physician comes in, the claims department is responsible for figuring out what to pay. As noted in Chapter 3, the same physician may be considered a PCP for one panel of members and a specialty physician for members not enrolled with that physician for primary care. Thus, the claims department must first determine if the service was provided by the submitting physician as a PCP or a specialty physician (based on whether recipient is a member of the physician's primary care panel). If the claim is considered a specialty care claim, then the claims department must find out whether the member's PCP authorized the service.

If the service was not authorized, the claims department must determine whether the member has already met his or her deductible (i.e., paid $200 out of pocket for other services before this claim was generated). If the deductible has not been met, the claims department applies some or all of the claim against the deductible, depending on the amount of the claim and the amount of previous claims. Assuming that the claim was for $100 and that no previous claims have been filed, the $100 goes against the $200 deductible, leaving only $100 for the member to pay out of pocket before coverage begins.

If the deductible has been met, the claims department must determine what to apply the 20-percent coinsurance against. If the physician who submitted the claim is a participating provider who has agreed to a fee schedule (see Chapter 3), then the percentage is applied against the maximum payment allowance. If the physician is not a participating provider, then the percentage is usually still applied against the maximum allowable charge, and the member is responsible for paying the difference.

If all the data have been received in a timely fashion and are accurate, the claim may be processed quickly and correctly. If, however, the member's enrollment file is not up to date (e.g., the member recently switched to a new PCP but the change was not captured electronically) or if the claim arrived before the authorization did (e.g., the claim was sent electronically but the mailed authorization arrived three days later), then the claim may be processed incorrectly. Therefore, the claims department must have processes in place to prevent these types of common errors from occurring.

Once a claim has been entered into the MCO's information systems, the processing occurs automatically. In many cases, a claims adjudicator (i.e., a claims clerk) will oversee the processing, but most of the activities are done without manual intervention.

Application of Medical Policies

In addition to managing the benefits an employer has purchased for its employees, the MCO must apply its policies regarding routine medical care and exceptions.

Routine Medical Policies

Routine medical policies are rules for using clinical information to make commonplace claims payment decisions. One policy might be to pay an assistant surgeon no more than 50 percent of the fee that the primary surgeon receives. Another might be to pay only for one abdominal procedure even if a surgeon bills for multiple procedures. For example, if the surgeon bills for both a hysterectomy (removal of the uterus) and a laparotomy (incision through the abdominal wall), the MCO would consider the two procedures to make up a single operation.

Medical Policies for Exceptions

Some medical policies pertain to payment for services that are not necessarily covered. Some exceptions, although uncommon, are relatively routine. For example, it is rare for MCOs to pay for cosmetic surgery, but they will pay for reconstructive surgery following trauma. Medical policies for exceptions also come into play when a claim arrives for a service that does not match up to the diagnosis the service is supposed to be for.

More difficult is the issue of experimental or investigational treatments. Until recently, no health plans paid for such treatments, but many lawsuits have compelled MCOs to pay for them even in the absence of clinical data supporting their use. The merits of such lawsuits are, for our purposes, beside the point, and strong arguments in support of any position on this issue can be constructed. What is to the point is that many state legislatures, as well as the federal government, have begun to apply a standard that requires coverage for investigational treatments undertaken as part of approved clinical research. When the demand for an experimental treatment does not take place in the context of an approved investigational program, all of the emotionally painful and scientifically difficult issues remain. In any case, the claims department's role is to pend the claim (hold it for further review) until the medical director is able to make a determination regarding coverage.

Pricing of Claims Payments

As noted earlier, the claims department must determine the appropriate amount to pay for each submitted claim. Chapter 3 mentioned that each MCO has a fee schedule for calculating the proper reimbursement for a procedure. If a participating provider submits a claim in excess of the maximum allowed in the fee schedule, the provider agrees (through his or her contract with the MCO) not to collect the difference between the claim and the maximum from either the MCO or the member. In some MCOs, however, the fee schedules for different plans differ from each other. For example, the fee schedule for the HMO may be higher or lower than the fee schedule for the PPO. The claims department must determine which schedule is in effect for each claim.

In the case of a claim from a nonparticipating provider (i.e., a provider that does not have a contract with the MCO), the claims department must still apply a maximum allowable fee, but the provider is free to bill the member the difference between that fee and the provider's charge.

Management of Claims Inventory

The number of claims received each day by an MCO is very high, and, depending on its size, the MCO may receive between 15,000 and 500,000 claims per month. These claims must all be accounted for and managed. Therefore, it is up to the claims department to put into place processes for logging each claim as it arrives, entering it into the information system, processing it correctly, and disposing of it (Figure 5–5). Most claims are disposed of by being paid, but claims can be adjusted or even denied.

It is easy for a claim to get lost in the sheer crush of volume. Therefore, the claims department, in conjunction with the mailroom, must ensure that every claim received through any means (U.S. Postal Service, fax, or e-mail) is immediately logged and entered into the system. Without logging and entry, claims would be impossible to track.

If the claims department processes claims with undue delay, several problems may arise. First, of course, providers and members will become unhappy. They have a right to ex-

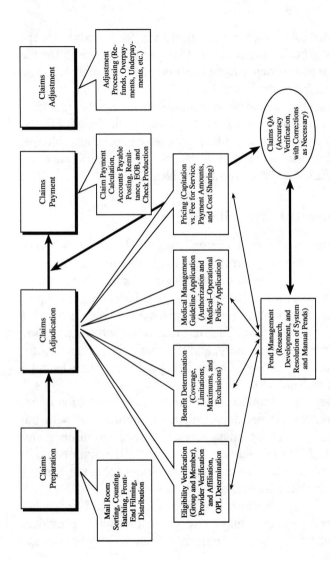

Figure 5–5 The claims management process. *Source:* Reprinted from R.L. McElfatrick and R.S. Eichler, Claims and Benefits Administration, in *Essentials of Managed Health Care*, 4th ed., F.R. Kongstvedt, ed., p. 496, © 2000, Aspen Publishers, Inc.

pect their claims to be processed quickly and efficiently. Further, if a backlog builds, providers are likely to send in duplicate claims in the belief (sometimes correct) that the original claims were lost. Duplicate claims add to the volume of claims that the MCO must deal with, and they increase the chance that an error will occur. For example, the MCO might wind up paying the second claim as well as the original and would then be faced with the task of collecting the overpayment from the provider who received it.

Many states, as well as large employers, have standards for how quickly a "clean claim" must be paid (a clean claim is a claim for which reasons to delay payment are absent). A clean claim usually must be paid in under 15 days, but sometimes only 7 days are allowed. Most MCO contracts with providers allow for up to 30 days for payment of a clean claim.

Claims that would be considered not clean include duplicate claims, claims for services that other parties may have primary responsibility for covering, and claims for nonauthorized services.

Management of Pended or Appealed Claims and Adjustments

When claims are pended, the claims department must have a system in place to make sure that they do not wind up in limbo. The department needs to track each pended claim and make sure that action ultimately is taken. Reasons that a claim might be pended include the need to allow the medical department to review the claim for medical necessity, confirm the member was eligible for services, or determine whether another party (e.g., another health insurance company) was primarily responsible for paying the claim.

Productivity and Quality Management

Productivity and quality management consists of activities intended to ensure that mistakes made in processing claims are kept to a minimum and that the claims department operates as efficiently as possible. Claims department managers measure how many claims a processor handlers per day, the accuracy (or conversely, the error rate) of the claims that are processed, the types of problems that occur with high frequency so that the cause of the problem may be addressed, and so forth. Managers of the claims department also look for ways to improve efficiency, such as using electronic imaging to capture paper documents, using electronic access to medical policy, and other labor-saving approaches. The greater the automation of the claims process, the higher the quality and efficiency of the process.

Other Party Liability

In some situations, more than one party is potentially liable to pay for a medical service. In the most common case, an individual is covered by two or more health policies, as happens when both members of a married couple are working and have employment-related health benefits. Unless each spouse took single coverage (i.e., coverage for the individual, not the entire family), two policies will be in force, and any children in the family will be covered twice over. Other party liability can also occur in cases where auto insurance comes into play (because the medical costs are associated with an auto accident) or where a government agency may be the primary insurer.

There are a complex set of rules that MCOs, health insurers, and other types of insurers follow in determining which one of several policies has primary payment responsibility and which policies are secondary. Benefits from two policies may also be available under certain circumstance. The same goes for benefits resulting from coverage through some type of government agency or department and from private insurance coverage. In all cases, a special function of the claims department is to deal with primary liability issues so that the MCO pays what it is supposed to but does not pay when another organization is obligated instead.

MEMBER SERVICES

The member services department acts as the interface between members and the MCO. In other words, when an individual member has a problem or needs assistance, it is member services that provides the necessary assistance. Member services is responsible for many functions, but only the most important are discussed here (see also Exhibit 5–1).

Provision of General Information

An MCO is in constant need of communicating with its members. The communication process begins before enrollment, when the MCO must provide information to prospective enrollees so they can make informed decisions, such as

Exhibit 5–1 Responsibilities of Member Services

Provide general information to members.
Provide routine communication to certain members.
Address member problems, complaints, appeals, and grievances.
Proactive outreach to members.
Perform continual surveillance and analysis of member satisfaction.

whether to join the plan and what PCP to select. It then continues throughout the enrollee's membership in the MCO and even beyond.

The MCO must routinely provide updated lists of participating providers, changes in hours of operations, changes in medical policies, and the like. It should also regularly offer educational information, such as health tips, immunization schedules, and smoking cessation and other forms of preventive medical education.

Routine Communication

Besides general information provided to all members, an MCO also needs to communicate specific information to certain members. Examples include the departure of a physician from the network and changes in the health benefits plan of a particular employer. In these cases, the member services department communicates the necessary information to any members who are affected by the change.

Some routine communications are required by law or regulation. For example, under the Employee Retirement Income Security Act (ERISA), an MCO must notify members leaving the health plan of their rights regarding continuation of coverage. It must also notify members about privacy and confidentiality, reimbursement policies, and appeal and grievance rights.

Addressing Member Problems, Complaints, Appeals, and Grievances

Working with members to manage problems, complaints, appeals, and grievances is perhaps the most important function performed by member services (Table 5–1). MCOs are required to address member problems and other issues under state and federal laws and regulations, although the specifics of the requirements vary from state to state.

Member problems range from something as simple as an incorrect identification card to something as complex as a

Table 5–1 Inquiries, Complaints, and Grievances

Measure	25th Percentile	Mean	75th Percentile
Inquiries per 1,000 MPM	133	150	142
Total complaints per 1,000 MPM	0.34	0.40	0.49
Total grievances per 1,000 MPM	0.16	0.32	0.43
Average complaint resolution time (days)	15.8	20.5	30.0
Average grievance resolution time (days)	29.9	39.3	44.1

MPM = members per month.
Courtesy of Ernst & Young LLP Proprietary Managed Care Benchmarking Study, 1997–1999, Washington, DC.

mishandled claim for medical expenses. MCOs have a special interest in helping members select physicians in an HMO or a POS plan and straightening out problems with authorization and other unique aspects of managed care.

Members have the right to file a formal complaint. Although a member may bring a complaint based on his or her first contact with the MCO (e.g., a complaint about rude or unprofessional behavior by a provider), most complaints stem from problems that are not resolved to the members' satisfaction. For example, an MCO may deny a medical claim on the grounds that the service in question is not covered, but the member might disagree.

All MCOs have rules and procedures in place for the resolution of complaints. The rules might require timelines for responding to a complaint (e.g., a response must be made within 30 days), require the existence of formal tracking mechanisms, and define who must review particular types of complaints and respond to them (e.g., the medical director might have to review all medically related complaints and the chief operating officer might be have to review all complaints about member services). The entire review process and all communications with the member are carefully documented.

An appeal is a formal request for review of a decision regarding coverage for specified medical costs or procedures. In most states, an appeal of a coverage decision requires an external review of the decision (the use of external reviews may be mandated by the federal government at some point as well). In an external review, physicians who are not employed by the MCO and are otherwise independent of it review the case and reach a determination. Again, detailed rules apply to an external review, and there is a timeline for the entire process. In some cases, a special "expedited review" is required—when the medical procedure is urgent (e.g., an experimental transplant). The conclusion reached by the review panel is usually binding on the MCO.

A grievance is a special type of formal complaint and requires a formal response by the MCO. The response must follow specific guidelines, although these tend to differ from state to state. Federal programs such as Medicare also have formal grievance procedures.

Grievances, as compared with other types of complaints, are especially likely to involve an external agency, usually a governmental one. A federal agency may be drawn in if the grievance is brought by an enrollee in Medicare or the Federal Employees Health Benefits Program, and the relevant state insurance department may be drawn in if the grievance is brought by an enrollee in a commercial insuance plan or HMO. The grievance procedures of a health plan self-funded by the employer must meet requirements mandated by ERISA.

Grievance procedures can differ from one type of coverage to another, but in all cases they include formal hearings and testimony (in the MCO, not a court of law) and have timeline and documentation requirements. If the grievance procedures do not result in an outcome satisfactory to the member, the member may still have recourse to an external agency or to the courts.

Proactive Outreach

If all that a member services department did was to handle problems, complaints, appeals, and grievances, it would not be filling its real potential. Proactively reaching out to members can have a powerful impact on member satisfaction and on the operations of the MCO. For instance, a welcoming call to new members can help them understand how the MCO operates, answer any questions they have, and take care of any issues that may have already arisen. Contacting members who have not extensively used the MCO's services is one way to make sure that they are satisfied with their membership.

Surveillance and Analysis of Member Satisfaction

An MCO must continually gauge the level of member satisfaction. Periodic surveys will allow the MCO to discover how members view their health plans and to pick up on trends early on. A survey may contain general questions intended to expose the overall level of satisfaction with the MCO or may contain narrow questions targeted at specific issues, such as the adequacy of the provider network. In some cases, formal member satisfaction surveys are compulsory (e.g., Medicare mandates their use). Further, in order to obtain external accreditation (see Chapter 7), an MCO must perform broad member satisfaction surveys and act on the results.

FINANCE AND UNDERWRITING

The finance and underwriting departments of an MCO are responsible for managing the money. The most important of their many functions are described below, after the following brief account of the financial measures used in MCOs.

Perhaps the most common unit of measure is per member per month (PMPM). To illustrate, suppose the finance department reports that the cost of the drug benefit for a particular health benefits plan is $20 PMPM. That means that on average the monthly cost for a member with that drug benefits plan is $20. The monthly cost for one particular member might be $300, it might be zero for another member, but it averages $20.

The other two measures—whole dollars and percent of premium—are even easier to understand. The first, whole dollars, is just what it sounds like—the total amount spent (or, in the case of income, the total amount received in the form of premium payments). The second measure, which is also what it sounds like, is easiest to understand in the context of reporting costs. For example, the cost of hospital care may represent 35 percent of each premium dollar (i.e., for each dollar of premium collected, $0.35 goes toward paying for hospital care). Whole dollars and percent of premium are usually reported for each month as well as for the year (or year to date).

The following illustrates various ways of reporting the same results. Assume that the MCO collects, in the form of premium payments, $175 PMPM, spends 35 percent of each dollar received on hospital care, and has 100,000 members covered under the health benefits plan. The amount collected equals $175 *PMPM*, $17,500,000 *per month* in whole dollars ($175 × 100,000), and $210,000,000 *per year* in whole dollars ($17,500,000 × 12). As for hospital costs, they equal 35 percent of the premium collected, or $61.25 *PMPM* ($175 × .35), $6,125,000 *per month* in whole dollars ($17,500,000 × .35), and $73,500,000 *per year* in whole dollars ($210,000,000 × .35)

Operational Finance

Operational finance refers to the overall functions of the finance department. The most important of these functions are to track all money that moves into and out of the MCO, track where it goes, identify how much goes where, and note why it does so. Following is a brief review of the major areas managed by the finance department.

Premium Revenue

The first step in the financial process is to receive the premium payments owed. These are actually accounted for by the finance department before the money arrives. The revenue at this point is referred to as *accrued revenue* or *booked revenue*; it is referred to as *cash revenue* after the actual receipt of the money. Why the difference? Because the MCO must know ahead of time how much money it expects to receive and to account for that money properly. Over time, the finance department (along with the billing and enrollment departments) must reconcile the amount of money paid by an employer (or government agency) against the amount the MCO believes it is owed based on the enrolled members. The total amount of premium owed is of course equal to the number of enrollees and the price of the health benefits plan.

Medical Costs

The next step is to determine where the money is to go. The majority of the money, between 80 and 95 percent in most cases, goes toward medical costs. As described elsewhere, there are many types of providers and medical services. It is up to the finance department to track how much money goes for each type of service and to each provider. For example, an MCO will usually track how much money is being spent on

- primary care
- specialty care
- hospital or other inpatient institutional care
- ambulatory surgery or outpatient procedures and diagnostics
- prescription drugs
- emergency or urgent care

The MCO will also usually track medical expenses by major line of business. For example, Medicare is tracked separately from commercial business; small group business, large group business, and self-insured business are tracked separately; and so forth.

Note that an MCO must book expenses for medical services well before it receives claims for those services. If the MCO were to book expenses only for already received claims, it would seriously miscalculate what the costs will eventually total. For instance, the costs of medical services are influenced by changes in membership numbers, the health benefits plans in force, and seasonality (medical costs vary depending on the season; e.g., little elective surgery is scheduled over Thanksgiving). The finance department must estimate what the costs are going to be and reserve enough money to pay for them.

An MCO puts aside money in a reserve—known as the IBNR (incurred but not reported)—to pay for medical claims that come in over time but about which it does not know any specifics.

There are numerous techniques that the finance department, with help from the actuarial and underwriting departments, uses to calculate the IBNR. The point here is that the finance department has the responsibility to ensure the MCO has put aside sufficient funds to pay for medical expenses.

Administrative Costs

Administrative costs fall into many categories. Common categories include

- marketing and sales
- member services
- medical management
- finance
- actuarial and underwriting
- legal
- claims
- enrollment and billing
- information systems

The Bottom Line

Lastly comes the bottom line. In almost all cases, MCOs, even nonprofit MCOs, are subject to taxation. Therefore, the cost of taxes must be taken into account. After that, the profit (in the case of a for-profit MCO) or reserve position (in the case of a nonprofit MCO) is reported.

Budgeting

All organizations require a budget in order to properly manage operations, and MCOs are no different. What makes budgeting for an MCO unique is the need to create a budget for medical expenses and a separate one for operational expenses. Further, different financial tools and techniques are used to create the two budgets. Budgeting, of course, is essential nonetheless, for it is only through the budget process that the MCO can test assumptions about how much to charge in premium or can determine what enhanced systems capabilities the MCO will be able to afford.

Reporting

Reporting is discussed apart from budgeting as there are several types of reporting that the finance department must do. It is the finance department that is usually responsible for creating reports for each employer, the U.S. Department of Labor, Medicare, and so forth, and sending them to the appropriate recipients.

Using special forms, the MCO must report financial and utilization results to the state insurance departments of those states in which it does business, although in some cases a state insurance department will accept the results that have been reported to the insurance department of the state the MCO is based in. Reporting these results is not an easy task, for the MCO must use a type of accounting based on statutory accounting principles (SAP) rather than the type based on generally accepted accounting principles (GAAP).* Each MCO must also produce an annual report containing both GAAP and SAP accounting information.

---

*The differences between SAP and GAAP are beyond the scope of this book.

Actuarial Services

The job of the actuarial services department is to estimate future medical expenses. The estimates are influenced by the design of the benefits plan, changes in laws (e.g., the mandating of certain benefits), the configuration of the network (e.g., fee schedules), assumptions about utilization patterns, and so forth. The actuarial services department also examines the IBRN calculations to ensure that an adequate amount of money has been set aside to pay for future medical claims.

Small and mid-sized MCOs may contract with external actuarial firms rather than hire staff actuaries. Even when an MCO does have staff actuaries, it is standard for outside actuaries to examine the IBNR and claims reserves as part of the annual audit.

Underwriting

Underwriting is related to estimating medical expenses, although it is done by nonactuaries. The two primary activities of the underwriting department are rate development and determining the level of risk of medical costs.

Rate Development

Underwriters are charged with using the cost estimates prepared by the finance and actuarial services departments to calculate the actual premium rates the MCO will charge customers. There are many types of rating, each useful in different circumstances. Following is a brief description of the most common.

Standard Community Rating. In this type of rating, an MCO creates a standard set of rates that it charges everyone regardless of differences in the size or makeup of the employer groups. For example, if the MCO determines that it needs $175 PMPM premium revenue, then it creates rates that will yield that amount, and that is what it charges. This does not mean there is a single monthly premium rate of $175 per person. The rate charged to a single individual is always higher than the premium revenue requirement, whereas family rates are usually lower than what they would be if each person were charged $175. The reason is that the medical costs for children are far less than for adults and that the administrative cost of enrolling a family is not that much higher than that of enrolling a single person. Standard community rating is often used in the small group market.

Adjusted Community Rating and Community Rating by Class. In adjusted community rating, an MCO calculates a standard community rate, then adjusts it based on a number of variables. The most common factors influencing the adjustment are the anticipated size of families and the proportion of families versus the proportion of single individuals. If families are small, then less revenue is needed for each family, for example. Another factor, though it is less commonly used, is the employer's type of business (certain types of businesses are considered higher risk than others).

Experience Rating. This type of rating reflects the actual medical experience of the employer group. If the group has had high medical expenses in the past, it will be charged a higher premium than a group whose medical costs have been low. Experience rating depends on the ability to differentiate between trends and just plain bad luck. For example, a group may have high expenses one year because of a single terrible auto accident. Another group's high expenses, on the other hand, may be due to the fact that all the employees and their families smoke asbestos while riding motorcycles under the influence of alcohol. The first group's history of high expenses was owing to bad luck and does not indicate that its expenses will remain high, whereas the high expenses of the second group are guaranteed to continue. Thus, experience rating is used only for groups with enough enrollees to allow the MCO to determine whether their history of medical costs reflects actual trends.

Rating for Self-Insured Employers. Even the account of a self-insured employer needs to have "rates" calculated so that the employer knows the likely future cost of employee health benefits and the employees can be charged for whatever portion is their responsibility. Although these are not true premium rates, they are often referred to as a "premium equivalent" since they perform much the same function.

Determining the Level of Risk

The other major activity of the underwriting department is to determine the level of risk of medical costs. Actuaries determine the overall risk of medical costs, but it is up to the underwriters to apply those principles to employer groups or individuals applying for health insurance coverage. The underwriters take many factors into account, including past medical claims history, current medical conditions, and so forth. In some cases, such as where open enrollment periods are mandated or in states that require MCOs to issue coverage to small groups regardless of their past history of costs, the underwriting department has little effect. Otherwise, when an employer seeks coverage from the MCO, the department analyzes the relevant factors and determines whether to offer coverage, what products to offer, and what rates to charge for those products.

INFORMATION SYSTEMS

An MCO's information system comprises the computer hardware and software and the telecommunications technologies it uses to store and transmit information. The overall information system will typically include a mainframe system to handle day-to-day operations, an internal network to allow electronic communication within the MCO, Internet or e-commerce capabilities for communication with the outside world, and telephone systems. It will also likely include private communications systems for business-to-business electronic interchange, data storage and analysis systems, and so forth.

The information system constitutes the backbone of the MCO's operations. All the activities described in this chapter and others depend on computer hardware and software, and if the information system is not working efficiently and properly, the MCO's ability to manage its finances, maintain membership data, process claims, and manage medical cases will be diminished. Therefore, the information system must be updated continually, and the various hardware and software problems that plague every MCO must be addressed promptly.

The MCO's ability to conduct business with other parties, such as providers and employers, also depends on its information system. Great quantities of paper are still used in the transaction of business, but paper is rapidly being replaced by electronic forms of information storage and transmission. Under the Health Insurance Portability and Accountability Act, the numerous conflicting standards for electronic transactions are being made more uniform, which will lead to even faster adoption of electronic transactions as the norm.

CONCLUSION

Although 83 to 95 percent of each dollar of premium is spent on clinical services, administrative activities make up most of what an MCO does. The MCO's normal functions include enrolling members, billing for and receiving premium payments, processing authorizations and other aspects of medical management, and paying claims. In addition, the MCO must ensure it has the means to help members resolve problems and manage complaints, appeals, and grievances. Finally, it must have the appropriate staff, as well as the appropriate information technologies, for managing its finances. Because of the complexity of its normal operations, the administrative challenges facing the typical MCO would be hard to overestimate.

CHAPTER 6

Medicare and Medicaid

LEARNING OBJECTIVES

- Understand the basic issues involved with Medicare managed care
- Understand key legal and regulatory issues in the government entitlement programs
- Understand the basic issues involved with Medicaid managed care
- Understand the historical roots of the Medicare and Medicaid programs, and how that applies to managed care
- Understand different types of organizational models to deliver services in the public sector

---

Managed care organizations (MCOs) offer services to a variety of market segments. The most important of these is the commercial market segment consisting of employers who offer health insurance or managed care coverage to their employees. A related segment is made up of individual purchasers of coverage, but individual coverage and group coverage operate in basically the same way (see Chapter 5 for an account of the differences). The focus of this chapter is on two noncommercial market segments—those composed of Medicare and Medicaid enrollees.

MEDICARE

Medicare, which began in 1965, is the most important health care entitlement program in the nation. It provides health care benefits for the elderly, for persons with end-stage renal disease (i.e., kidney failure), and for some disabled persons. It has traditionally operated as a fee-for-service program. Typically, the federal government contracts with fiscal intermediaries (e.g., nongovernment organizations such as Blue Cross and Blue Shield plans) to process Medicare claims (in other words, providers bill the fiscal intermediaries for services received by Medicare beneficiaries). The fee-for-service component of Medicare is often referred to as "traditional Medicare," to differentiate it from the managed care component. Traditional Medicare has a rigid schedule of maximum fees based on the resource-based relative value scale for professionals (see Chapter 3) and a variety of payment mechanisms for hospitals, nursing homes, ambulatory surgical centers, and so forth.

Beginning in 1985, Medicare allowed MCOs to offer services. Medicare beneficiaries were able to enroll in health maintenance organizations (HMOs) and were treated like commercial members, although the HMOs were subject to special rules regarding sales and marketing, reporting, and reimbursement. Later, the Balance Budget Act of 1997 (BBA) expanded the benefits options and the plans available under Medicare, which now include Medicare HMOs or HMO-like organizations. Medicare managed care now goes by the title Medicare+Choice.

Medicare managed care is generally a pure retail market segment. In other words, MCOs that offer Medicare products do so, not on a group basis, but on an individual basis. (There are exceptions—some HMOs offer Medicare coverage to retirees through their former employers, for instance—but these are unimportant for the purposes of this chapter.) A Medicare beneficiary can choose to enroll in any Medicare+Choice plan in the local area and can choose to drop out as well. Until the BBA, Medicare beneficiaries in Medicare+Choice plans had the right to join and drop out at will; however, the new regulations, after a phase-in period, will require a Medicare+Choice beneficiary enrolled in a plan to remain with the plan for a set period of time (up to nine months). The "lock in" provision allows for exceptions based on a variety of reasons (e.g., the Medicare+Choice plan exits the market or the enrollee moves to another locale).

In general, Medicare beneficiaries find Medicare+Choice plans attractive because they offer benefits beyond those available in traditional Medicare. One such benefit that is commonly offered is (limited) coverage for prescription drugs. Another is coverage for preventive services. Medicare+Choice plans also reduce or eliminate deductibles and coinsurance, enhancing beneficiaries' access to care.

Medicare+Choice Managed Care Plans

Traditional Medicare HMOs

Traditional Medicare HMOs are similar to the Medicare managed care plans that existed prior to the BBA. They are licensed by the state (see Chapter 7 for a discussion of state licensure) or at least are subject to oversight by the state (e.g., a Medicaid-only HMO that is not licensed as a commercial HMO but still meets state oversight requirements). In essence, the Centers for Medicare & Medicaid Services* (CMS) has delegated the oversight of commercial and Medicaid HMOs to the states and accepts state certification as sufficient evidence that an HMO is meeting financial and market conduct standards. In fact, CMS has delegated to the states the authority to decide what types of MCO can enter into a Medicare+Choice contract.

Besides the relevant state requirements, Medicare+Choice HMOs face additional federal requirements. As one example, the Balanced Budget Act of 1997 requires that an MCO have at least 5,000 members (or 1,500 members if operating in a rural area) in order to secure a Medicare+Choice contract. Other federal requirements are discussed toward the end of the chapter.

Provider-Sponsored Organizations

Provider-sponsored organizations (PSOs) are similar to HMOs except that they are owned and operated by the providers themselves. The BBA defines a PSO as an organization most of whose services are provided by the sponsoring providers (i.e., providers with majority ownership or control of the organization) or by affiliated providers (i.e., providers at direct or indirect financial risk for the organization). In particular, in an urban area, 70 percent of health care services (as measured by expenditures) must be provided directly by the sponsoring providers or by affiliated providers (the required

---

*Called the Health Care Financing Administration (HCFA) until July 1, 2001.

proportion is only 60 percent in a rural area). For organizations that meet the Act's definition of a PSO, the minimum number of precontract enrollees required is reduced to 1,000 (500 in a rural area), and this requirement may also be waived.

PSOs were created under the BBA and pertain solely to Medicare+Choice. They may be licensed by the state, in which case they are functionally similar to HMOs, but state licensure is not always required. If a state does not license a PSO, the PSO can apply for a waiver from CMS to become licensed to enroll Medicare+Choice members though not commercial or Medicaid members. Waivers of this type are supposed to expire in 2002.

PSOs are not required to meet the same solvency standards as state-licensed HMOs. Whereas both HMOs and PSOs must maintain defined levels of liquidity (i.e., cash or cash-equivalent funds) and defined levels of reserves (i.e., money set aside for financially difficult times), the levels required of an HMO are higher than for a PSO. The thinking behind not requiring PSOs to maintain the higher levels is that the providers in a PSO are themselves at risk for services and do not need to worry as much about paying for services to others.

When the BBA was passed, providers greeted the opportunity to create PSOs with enthusiasm. Unfortunately, relatively few PSOs ever got off the ground, and most of those that did lost significant amounts of money. Most of the PSOs created as part of an initial demonstration project went out of existence, and new applicants for PSO status did not finalize the process and become operational. Although PSO status remains an option under Medicare+Choice, at the time of this writing few PSOs are in operation.

Preferred Provider Organizations

Preferred provider organizations (PPOs), along with HMOs and PSOs, are defined as coordinated care plans by the BBA. Before the Act, a PPO offered by an indemnity insurer might not have been able to enter into a Medicare risk contract because it was not an HMO or an HMO-like MCO. The BBA loosened the requirements for participating in Medicare+ Choice, and now the only stipulation is that a PPO—or any entity wishing to have an Medicare+Choice contract—be licensed as a risk-bearing entity by the state and that its members be individuals "who are receiving health benefits through the organization," regardless of the exact nature of the risk arrangement. As noted above, the state determines whether the type of license held by a PPO, a PPO sponsor, an HMO, or any other risk-bearing entity should enable the organization to enter into a contract with CMS and assume risk for the comprehensive range of Medicare services.

Point-of-Service Plans

Under Medicare+Choice, HMOs may offer a point-of-service (POS) benefit to their Medicare enrollees. In general, a point-of-service benefit allows an enrollee to receive services delivered by extra-network providers, although the services, while still covered, are subject to a higher deductible and a higher co-pay. The regulations provide great latitude in the design of the benefit, how it is financed (e.g., it could be offered as an additional benefit funded by Medicare capitation payments), the charges to enrollees, and the extent of its availability (e.g., it could be restricted to employer group retirees).

However, organizations offering a POS option are subject to additional monitoring by the CMS to ensure continued compliance with standards pertaining to financial solvency, availability and accessibility of care, quality assurance, member appeals, and marketing.

Private Fee-for-Service Plans

An organization may choose to enter into a contract with CMS to offer a private health insurance plan that reimburses providers on a fee-for-service basis and does not limit enrollees to the use of network providers. As an enrollee of a Medicare+Choice private fee-for-service (PFFS) plan, a Medicare beneficiary may use any Medicare-participating provider who agrees to provide services to the beneficiary, and the organization sponsoring the PFFS plan (e.g., a private insurer) will pay for covered services in a manner similar to a traditional indemnity plan operating in the private marketplace. A PFFS plan may not pay its providers other than on a fee-for-service basis and may not place providers at financial risk for the utilization of services.

PFFS plans are rather elaborate, and at the time of this writing, relatively rare. To illustrate this complexity, a basic description of a PFFS follows:

> The PFFS plan may have a network of providers who agree to the terms of the plan, but the law also provides for "deemed" participating providers. A provider is deemed to be a participating provider if he or she (or the entity) is aware of the beneficiary's enrollment in the PFFS plan, and the provider is

aware of, or has been given a reasonable opportunity to be made aware of, the terms and conditions of payment under the plan "in a manner reasonably designed to effect informed agreement" to participate, as stated in the regulations. A non-contracting provider may only receive, in total payments (from the PFFS plan and from enrollee cost sharing), an amount equal to what would have been paid in total under original Medicare. Contracting and deemed providers may also receive additional payments from the enrollee ("balance billing") up to 15% of the PFFS plan payment amount. The PFFS organization is charged with ensuring that providers adhere to the limits on permissible balance billed amounts; failure to monitor adherence to the requirement can result in [CMS's] decision not to renew the organization's contract. Enrollees may incur additional liability if the PFFS retrospectively denies coverage (as not Medicare-covered, or for non-Medicare-covered benefits not covered under the plan).*

REIMBURSEMENT OF MEDICARE+CHOICE MCOs

CMS's method of reimbursing Medicare+Choice MCOs for services is complicated. (As noted in Chapter 5, the pricing and premium payment methods used by commercial products

---

*Quoted from C. Zarabozo and J. LeMasurier, "Medicare and Managed Care," in *The Managed Health Care Handbook,* 4th ed., ed. P.R. Kongstvedt (Gaithersburg, MD, Aspen Publishers, 2000), 1060–1085.

are complicated as well.) In calculating the proper reimbursement, CMS uses historical costs for Medicare services in the same service area as the MCO to arrived at a computed amount, which is then usually reduced by 5 percent and adjusted further to account for enrollees who are sicker or healthier than expected. A detailed explanation of the method is both beyond the scope of the book and would be of doubtful value, as the rules keep changing. For example, various approaches to adjusting for severity of illness are being challenged, and it is not possible to say with certainty what approach will be used in the long term. Therefore, interested readers should go directly to CMS for information (a good place to start is the Web site www.cms.gov). Also, a thorough discussion of the method used is found in the *Managed Health Care Handbook.*

Note that Medicare+Choice MCOs may charge enrollees an additional premium for benefits not covered under traditional Medicare. Historically, Medicare HMOs did not charge Medicare enrollees for drug coverage, for instance, or for the elimination of a deductible or coinsurance. The savings from managed care paid for these added benefits. However, as payments to HMOs from HCFA (CMS) came under pressure as HCFA began to reduce or failed to sufficiently increase payments to HMOs, many HMOs did begin to charge Medicare+Choice members an additional premium.

SPECIAL REQUIREMENTS FOR
MEDICARE+CHOICE MCOs

As noted earlier, the main Medicare+Choice participation requirement for MCOs is licensure by the state (PSOs, under limited conditions, are excepted from this requirement). CMS, however, has many additional requirements, the most important of which are described below.

Quality Standards

To gain state licensure, MCOs must meet certain quality standards, but the standards vary widely from state to state. To gain accreditation (see Chapter 7), MCOs must meet more rigorous quality standards. To participate in Medicare+Choice, they must meet standards similar to those used by accreditation programs as well as some special standards. Medicare+Choice MCOs are required to

- have an ongoing quality assessment and performance improvement program that focuses on health outcomes and measurable change
- use peer review for quality assurance purposes
- use standardized measures as well as the following information-gathering tools:
  1. Health Plan Employer Data Information Set (HEDIS® provides information about service and quality)
  2. Quality Improvement System for Managed Care (QISMC contains standards to be used by Medicare and Medicaid health plans)
  3. Consumer Assessment of Health Plans Survey (CAHPS)
  4. Health Outcomes Survey (HOS)
- have written procedures for remedial action to correct problems
- undergo external review by peer review organizations

Except for HEDIS, which is briefly discussed in Chapter 7, none of the tools listed above is covered in this book. For information about them, consult the *Managed Health Care Handbook* or go to www.cms.gov.

Limitations on Physician Incentive Plans

The BBA prohibits certain types of financial incentives for physicians participating in a Medicare+Choice plan, specifically payments "made directly or indirectly under the plan to a physician or physician group as an inducement to reduce or limit medically necessary services provided with respect to a specific individual enrolled with the organization."

The Act also provides that certain requirements must be met in the event that physicians or physician groups are placed at "substantial" financial risk for services they do not directly render. In particular, the MCO must provide stop-loss protection for the providers (see Chapter 3) and conduct periodic satisfaction surveys of current and former enrollees (this requirement can be met by using the CAHPS survey mentioned in the preceeding bullet list). The Act sets out specifics for the stop-loss insurance and defines what is to be considered substantial financial risk. To oversimplify, physicians or physician groups are considered to be at substantial risk if over 25 percent of their potential payments are at risk.

Each year, every Medicare+Choice MCO must provide descriptive information about its physician incentive plan in sufficient detail to enable CMS to determine whether the plan complies with the provisions of the BBA. It must also disclose to Medicare beneficiaries, upon request, whether it uses a physician incentive plan, the types of incentives used, and whether it provides stop-loss protection. In addition, if the MCO was required to conduct a survey, it must provide a summary of the results to Medicare beneficiaries upon request.

Access Standards

CMS (then called HCFA) established Medicare+Choice requirements regarding access to care under the BBA as well as through an executive order from President Clinton relating to the Consumer Bill of Rights and Responsibilities. The stipulations include

- requiring unrestricted communication between patients and health care professionals through the prohibition of "gag" clauses (i.e., the contract between a physician and the MCO cannot prohibit the physician from giving the patient any medical advice);
- using the "prudent layperson" (i.e., a person who is not a medical professional) definition of what constitutes an emergency, the liability of the Medicare+Choice organization for the cost of such care, and a requirement to cover appropriate maintenance and post-stabilization care after an emergency;
- covering out-of-area dialysis during an enrollee's temporary absence from the service area;
- limiting co-payments for emergency services to no more than $50;
- specifying that the decision of the examining physician treating the individual enrollee prevails regarding when the enrollee may be considered stabilized for discharge or transfer;

- requiring plans to permit women enrollees to choose direct access to a women's health specialist within the network for women's routine and preventive health;
- requiring plans to have procedures approved by CMS for identification of individuals with complex or serious medical conditions, assessment of such individuals, and development of an appropriate treatment plan, including the right to direct access to specialists under the treatment plan; and
- requiring that services be provided in a "culturally competent" manner (i.e., with sensitivity towards cultural, ethnic, and language differences).

Member Appeals

Medicare+Choice enrollees have the right to an administrative and judicial appeals process regulated by CMS rather than the state insurance department. Medicare appeals rules apply to decisions regarding the coverage or cost of an item or a service included in the Medicare contract (Medicare-covered items and services as well as additional and supplemental benefits), including payment for out-of-network services received in an emergency.

The appeals process includes an internal review of the disputed decision. In addition, the enrollee can demand the decision be subjected to an external review by an entity under contract to CMS. If this entity upholds the original decision, then, for claims valued at $100 or more, the enrollee can demand a review of the decision by an administrative law judge. If the judge rules in favor of the enrollee, the Medicare+Choice MCO does not have the right of appeal. If judge rules against the enrollee, the enrollee can demand a review of the decision by the Departmental Appeals Board of the U.S. Department of Health and Human Services. For claims valued at $1,000 or more, the enrollee can also demand a judicial review of the decision in federal court.

The Medicare+Choice MCO must make the first-level determination "as expeditiously as the enrollee's health condition requires" but no later than 14 days from the date of the request. A reconsideration decision (by the organization or the review entity) must be made within 30 days. For expedited appeals, the standard is that a decision must be rendered within 72 hours.

Sales and Marketing

As mentioned earlier, Medicare+Choice MCOs market and sell their products to individual Medicare beneficiaries, and a beneficiary's decision to join an MCO is based on purely personal reasons. CMS has created many rules for market conduct, however, such as the following:

- The MCO must market throughout the entire service area in a nondiscriminatory manner.
- All marketing materials, including membership and enrollment materials, must be approved by CMS before use.
- Prospective enrollees must be given sufficient descriptive materials to allow them to make an informed decision regarding enrollment.
- Prospective enrollees must be given a summary of benefits form that uses standard definitions of benefits and a standardized format.

Examples of sales and marketing activities that are prohibited by CMS include

- door-to-door solicitation
- discriminatory marketing (e.g., avoiding low-income areas)
- misleading marketing or misrepresentation
- offering monetary incentives as an inducement to enroll
- completing any portion of the enrollment application for a prospective enrollee

Corporate Compliance

Corporate compliance activities are directed toward (1) ensuring the organization conforms to legal and regulatory requirements and (2) preventing and detecting illegal behavior. CMS, through the Office of the Inspector General (OIG), created guidelines that a Medicare+Choice MCO must follow. When evaluating a corporate compliance program, the OIG considers whether the elements listed in Exhibit 6–1 are present in the organization.

For a corporate compliance program to be effective, the following are required:

- creation of a special compliance committee
- designation of a corporate compliance officer
- creation of standards of conduct for employees
- creation of policies and procedures specifically designed to ensure compliance with the Medicare+Choice rules
- special training for employees

Exhibit 6-1 Office of the Inspector General Corporate Compliance Guidance

1. The development and distribution of written standards of conduct, as well as written policies and procedures, that promote the organization's commitment to compliance and that address specific areas of potential fraud.
2. The designation of a chief compliance officer and other appropriate bodies, e.g., a corporate compliance committee, charged with the responsibility of operating and monitoring the compliance program and who report directly to the CEO and the governing body.
3. The development and implementation of regular, effective education and training programs for all affected employees.
4. The development of effective lines of communication between the compliance officer and all employees, including a process, such as a hotline, to receive complaints (and the adoption of procedures to protect the anonymity of complainants and to protect callers from retaliation).
5. The use of audits or other risk evaluation techniques to monitor compliance and assist in the reduction of identified problem areas.
6. The development of disciplinary mechanisms to consistently enforce standards and the development of policies addressing dealings with sanctioned and other specified individuals.
7. The development of policies to respond to detected offenses and to initiate corrective action to prevent similar offenses.

Source: Reprinted from Final Compliance Program Guidance for Medicare+Choice Organizations, 64 *Federal Register* 61893; November 15, 1999.

- employee surveys that focus on compliance issues
- a "hotline" for employees to report violations of the Medicare+Choice rules
- exit interviews of employees in which possible rule violations are enquired about

- audits of compliance
- screening for individuals or entities barred from participation in federal programs (applies to employees, providers, and vendors)
- creation of an internal investigation program that focuses on Medicare+Choice rule violations

MEDICAID

At the same time that Medicare was created in 1965, an additional program was created to provide health insurance coverage for low-income individuals—Medicaid. Unlike Medicare, Medicaid is administered by the states, though half of the funding comes from the federal government. Policies, rules, and regulations pertaining to eligibility, coverage, payment, and services vary from state to state. Recent national legislation, including the Americans with Disabilities Act, welfare reform legislation, the BBA, and the State Children's Health Insurance Program, have also had a direct impact on Medicaid.

Medicaid provides coverage primarily for three groups:

1. Low-income individuals, mostly healthy women and children, make up 70 percent of Medicaid enrollees.
2. Aged and younger persons who have a chronic illness or condition and are disabled make up the second largest group.
3. Institutionalized individuals, who make up the third group, are really a subset of the second group. This population includes persons in nursing homes or spe-

cialized facilities for the developmentally disabled or mentally retarded.

The second two groups, despite representing a minority of the Medicaid enrollees, are responsible for the vast majority of Medicaid costs. It is the first group, however, that has been the primary focus of Medicaid managed care, since these individuals are most similar to the commercial population and therefore more easily integrated into managed care programs.

Like Medicare, Medicaid was operated as a fee-for-service program, and providers billed Medicaid for services rendered. Physicians are not required to participate in the Medicaid program (i.e., agree to accept Medicaid reimbursement as payment in full), and many do not. Hospitals are not required to participate unless they are nonprofit; however, almost all hospitals participate regardless.

Because Medicaid now consumes a very large portion of each state's budget, states are looking for ways to control the cost of the program. For the most part, to achieve this goal states have used the strategy of paying very low fees to providers. Although partially successful as a way of moderating cost increases, this strategy, in some cases, has also had the unintended effect of obstructing access to care, since many providers are unwilling to accept Medicaid patients in return for low levels of reimbursement.

An additional problem facing state Medicaid programs is that coordination of care for Medicaid enrollees has often been lacking. To address this problem and meet the goal of controlling cost without reducing access, the states have turned to managed care. To implement managed care programs, the states have required waivers (i.e., permission) from the federal government, since Medicaid was originally developed as a fee-for-service system. The necessary waivers have been routinely granted. At this time, most states have created Medicaid managed care programs and have seen positive results both for cost management and improved access and coordination of health care.

There are a variety of Medicaid managed care programs. Some look much like traditional HMOs. In one model, the so-called primary care case manager model, Medicaid members use primary care physicians to coordinate care, but other HMO features, such as financial risk sharing, are absent. A few states have made enrollment in managed care mandatory for low-income Medicaid recipients. Some states use commercial HMOs to offer services, others have chartered Medicaid-only MCOs, while many states actually run their own managed care programs.

Marketing to the Medicaid population is a specialized function. Certain activities, such as door-to-door solicitation, are generally prohibited. Cultural diversity is a highly important issue in Medicaid, including the need to accommodate non-English-speaking individuals. Because of the low educational levels prevalent in some Medicaid populations, materials that explain the program have to be written in easy-to-understand language. At least half the states with Medicaid managed care programs use "information brokers" to help poorly educated Medicaid beneficiaries access the system.

States monitor the activities of Medicaid MCOs in much the same way that the federal government monitors the activities of Medicare HMOs. One particularly important measurement tool is HEDIS, which is discussed in Chapter 7.

CONCLUSION

Medicare and Medicaid, as entitlement health care programs at the federal and state levels, together represent enormous expenditures of tax dollars. Medicare, by implementing managed care, has been able to improve its health care benefits while keeping costs reasonable. State Medicaid programs have successfully used managed care to control costs and enhance the coordination of care, which explains why most states have incorporated managed care into their Medicaid programs. Because Medicare and Medicaid are government programs and have widely different characteristics, MCOs that undertake to serve Medicare and Medicaid populations must be prepared to modify their operations to meet the programs' special requirements.

CHAPTER 7

Regulation and Accreditation in Managed Care

LEARNING OBJECTIVES

- Understand the basic issues involved with state regulation of managed care
- Understand the key components of the Employee Retirement Income Security Act
- Understand the key components of the Health Insurance Portability and Accountability Act
- Understand the key components of external accreditation of managed care organizations

---

Managed care is heavily regulated but the regulation is far from uniform. For most aspects of managed care, the states are responsible for regulating managed care organizations (MCOs). However, state regulation applies only to the provision of medical services insured by an MCO (i.e., services for which the MCO accepts the risk for medical expenses). If an employer retains the risk for medical expenses and the MCO simply provides administrative services, the state has less authority and the provision of medical services is regulated under a federal law entitled the Employee Retirement Income Security Act (ERISA). As a practical matter, most MCOs, because they have insured and self-insured accounts, are regulated by both the states and under ERISA. Further, as indicated above, some elements of state regulation do apply to the provision of medical care by self-insured employers.

Recently, a new federal law, the Health Insurance Portability and Accountability Act of 1996 (HIPAA), placed requirements and regulatory responsibilities on almost all elements of the health care system, including providers and MCOs, regardless of any other state or federal regulation. At this writing, the long debate at the federal level regarding a so-called patient's bill of rights has not yet reached an outcome.

This chapter briefly describes the regulation of MCOs by the states as well as the requirements set by HIPAA and ERISA. The reader should bear in mind that laws are always changing and that only very recent sources should be relied on for information about the regulations that pertain to MCOs.

STATE REGULATION

MCOs usually are regulated by more than one state agency. In almost all cases, the department of insurance regulates health maintenance organizations (HMOs), although some exceptions exist (e.g., in California, HMOs are regulated separately). In most states, the department of health also regulates HMOs. Insurance regulators assume principal responsibility for the financial aspects of HMO operations and, in many states, for external review of adverse benefit determinations. Health regulators focus on quality-of-care issues, utilization patterns, and the ability of participating providers to deliver adequate care. Preferred provider organizations (PPOs) are generally regulated by the department of insurance.

The National Association of Insurance Commissioners (NAIC), which represents insurance departments in the 50 states and the U.S. territories, created the HMO Model Act in 1972 as an archetype for legislation authorizing the establishment of HMOs and provide for an ongoing regulatory monitoring system. This model act, either in whole or in part, has now been enacted by 30 states and the District of Columbia. The remaining states also have adopted laws regulating HMOs, but these laws are not based on NAIC's HMO Model Act. The NAIC has also created other model acts for PPOs and utilization review organizations as well as for issues such as privacy, external review, and so forth. None of these model acts has the force of law, but each may be used by states in creating their own laws and regulations.

Licensure

The most important type of state regulation of MCOs is licensure. The license, usually termed a certificate of authority (COA), sets out the requirements that the MCO must meet in order to do business in the state. The many requirements for licensure include

- financial solvency (i.e., the MCO must have sufficient money to reliably pay claims)
- an adequate network
- adequate access to care, including uninterrupted access to emergency services
- an acceptable utilization management program
- an acceptable quality management program
- an acceptable member grievance program

- a provider credentialing verification system
- adequate information for members
- benefits plans that meet state requirements
- proper forms for groups
- proper forms for enrollees
- conversion rights for disenrolling members (i.e., some members who lose group coverage have the right to convert to an individual policy)

The exact nature of these requirements vary depending on the type of MCO, and some requirements may not apply under certain conditions (e.g., solvency requirements may not apply to a PPO that does not bear financial risk for medical expenses).

In addition to granting a license to an MCO, the state monitors the MCO's performance on a regular basis. For monitoring purposes, the state requires the MCO to provide quarterly financial reports and audited annual financial statements. If state officials believe that the MCO is not performing well (e.g., if it appears to be running low on money), they may intensify their scrutiny. In the most extreme circumstances, such as when bankruptcy appears imminent, the state insurance department may even seize control of the MCO to protect the interests of the covered members.

A third-party administrator (TPA) is an organization that administers group benefits and claims for a self-funded company or group. It usually does not assume any insurance risk. About two-thirds of the states require licensure of TPAs, and about one-third exempt TPAs from state licensure if they administer only single-employer, self-funded plans. State TPA laws typically govern the following:

- the TPA's written agreement with each insurer (which must include a statement of duties)
- the payment methodology
- the maintenance and disclosure of records
- insurer responsibilities, such as the determination of benefit levels
- the TPA's fiduciary obligations (e.g., in the collecting of charges and premiums)
- the issuance of TPA licenses and grounds for suspension or revocation
- the filing of annual reports
- the payment of fees

In addition to licensing health plans, many states require additional licensure or certification for utilization management activities that an MCO or TPA undertakes. Under NAIC's Utilization Review Model Act, HMOs, PPOs, freestanding medical management organizations, and other health care organizations that are subject to state regulation and provide or perform utilization review services are required to

- use documented clinical review criteria based on sound clinical evidence
- ensure that qualified health professionals administer the utilization review program
- abide by strict time limits for utilization review decisions

The model act prohibits compensation arrangements that encourage utilization review staff to make inappropriate determinations and provides for a process of appealing adverse decisions.

Regulation of Insured Business

Many laws and regulations apply to MCOs that are at risk for medical expenses and are not just providing administrative services. Some of the more common types are described below. The creation (and occasional removal) of these laws and regulations is influenced by politics, and thus they differ widely from state to state. As noted earlier, the provision of medical services by self-insured employers is governed by the provisions of ERISA (discussed in a later section) and is generally outside the scope of these laws and regulations. In fact, many employers self-insure primarily to avoid having their benefits plans subject to these laws and regulations.

Benefits Plans and Premium Rates

Every state requires MCOs to file benefits plans and premium rates. Some states require MCOs to obtain approval before offering benefits plans, others simply require notification. State rules that determine how MCOs may create premium rates also vary (as stated in Chapter 5, community rating may be required for small groups). It is common for an MCO to file a benefits plan in which some options are offered to enrollees, such as three different levels of copayment for physician visits. In filing the benefits plan, the MCO indicates what the options are.

Mandated Benefits

Most states have laws mandating certain benefits (e.g., mental health benefits and substance abuse benefits). If a benefit has been mandated, all MCOs and health insurance products must offer that benefit. Some states have many mandated benefits, others have relatively few. Some state laws mandating benefits also contain provisions directing how the benefits are to be applied. In the most common example, a state law might set a mandatory length of stay, such as two days, for the delivery of a baby, in which case an MCO may not discharge a newborn and mother in less than two days.

Provider-MCO Relationships

Some states have laws regulating the relationship between MCOs and providers. For instance, "any willing provider" laws, which are especially common, require an MCO to contract with any provider who meets credentialing criteria and is willing to accept the terms and conditions of the MCO's provider contract. In some states, "any willing provider" laws apply to pharmacies as well. Recently, a few states have passed laws regarding due process; these laws regulate how an MCO may terminate a contract with a provider. Prompt payment laws, which delineate how quickly an MCO must process claims and pay providers, are also common.

Provider Access

Access to certain types of providers has been legally protected in some states. For instance, laws giving women the right to access Ob/Gyns directly without having to go through a primary care provider are common. A few states have also passed laws allowing direct access to other types of providers, such as chiropractors, and a few have passed laws requiring an MCO to create a "standing authorization" for specialty physician services for certain clinical conditions. As for access to emergency services, most states require an MCO to use a "prudent layperson" standard in determining whether to pay for emergency care. In other words, if a normal nonclinically trained person would have been convinced that a true emergency existed, then the MCO must pay for the care.

External Appeals

Most states have adopted policies giving enrollees a right to appeal a denial of coverage and bring the issue before an external review entity, such as a private, state-approved organization. Although these policies differ widely, the right to an external review generally applies to denials of coverage that are based on medical necessity criteria or a determination that the services are experimental or investigational. In addition, these policies often contain provisions such as the following:

- The internal appeals process must be completed before the external review can be initiated.
- The plan must select an independent review entity from a list approved by the state or by a state official (typically the insurance commissioner).
- The external review entity must not be subject to a conflict of interest.
- The plan must pay the costs of the external review process.
- The external review entity's decision is to be binding on the plan.

Privacy

In recent years, state laws protecting the privacy of health care information have become popular. HIPAA also has provisions protecting the privacy and security of health information, but it allows states to pass stricter laws and regulations.

Health Plan Liability

In the past, a particular provision of ERISA limited the legal liability of insurance companies and health plans and effectively prevented enrollees from obtaining significant punitive damage awards from tort suits (i.e., lawsuits claiming damages). If a health plan or an insurance company did not act in bad faith, then the most that a plaintiff could recover was the insurance benefit itself. Certainly, some lawsuits resulted in large damage awards, but such awards were difficult to obtain. Many states have recently passed laws that increase the liability of health plans and insurance companies and make them subject to punitive damages in lawsuits. The issue of liability is the subject of intense ongoing debate at the federal level, since ERISA is a federal law.

Multi-State Operations

MCOs operating in more than one state must comply with the regulations of each state. It is usual for a state to require "foreign" HMOs (i.e., HMOs licensed in a different state) to meet the same requirements that apply to "domestic" HMOs. It is also possible for a state to require foreign HMOs to register to do business under the appropriate foreign corporation law and appoint an agent in the state for receipt of legal notifications.

Some states permit regulators who are considering the application of a foreign HMO to accept financial reports and other information from the HMO's state of origin, often referred to as the state of domicile. The NAIC also has established guidelines for coordinating examinations of HMOs licensed in more than one state. The coordinated examination is called for by the HMO's state of domicile; other states where the HMO operates are encouraged to participate. Occasionally, regulations in one state may hinder the operations of an HMO licensed in another state.

Historically, group insurance policies generally have been subject to the laws of the state of issuance (i.e., the state where the policies were originally issued). This general rule has been overtaken by the application of each state's insurance laws. In other words, it is usual for a state to require that any state resident covered under a group health policy issued in a different state receive the same coverage that would have been required had the group policy been issued within the state.

THE HEALTH INSURANCE PORTABILITY AND ACCOUNTABILITY ACT

HIPAA is a highly significant federal act whose provisions are being defined even as this chapter is being written. Passed in 1996 by a Republican congress and signed into law by a Democratic president, HIPAA is the most far-reaching federal health law since Medicare and Medicaid were passed in 1965. It also represents the first direct intrusion of the federal government into the regulation of insurance. As pointed out in the section above, states regulate insurance whereas the federal government regulates self-insured benefits plans. The provisions of HIPAA apply equally to insured and self-insured health benefits plans. However, HIPAA does not preempt state law provisions that are more stringent than the corresponding provisions in HIPAA, except in one area—electronic transaction standards (discussed below).

Portability and Access

HIPAA establishes standards for group health plans and group health insurance coverage that are intended to enhance access to health coverage. For HIPAA, a group health plan is an employer- or union-sponsored employee benefit plan (as defined in ERISA) that provides medical care through insurance, reimbursement, or otherwise. The health insurance issuer might be an insurance company, an insurance service organization, or an HMO.

HIPAA addresses the issue of preexisting medical conditions. It states that enrollment cannot be denied to individuals with preexisting medical conditions, nor can waiting periods be applied to the provision of services for these individuals based on their having these conditions. HIPAA also prohibits charging different premium rates to people within the same health benefits plan based solely on their medical conditions. HIPAA does not actually require any particular benefits (with a few exceptions noted later in this section). In other words, HIPAA does not dictate plan benefit design but does ensure greater access to group insurance.

HIPAA contains provisions that pertain to the guaranteed renewability of group health insurance as well as certain forms of health insurance portability. With regards to renewability, if a small employer (i.e., an employer with between 2 and 50 employees) has an insured health benefits plan with an insurance carrier, the employer has the right to renew its coverage with the carrier. In fact, HIPAA goes so far as to require insurance companies to guarantee access to their most common small group products to any small employers who seek them.

With regards to portability, individuals have the right to extend their health insurance coverage with an insurer if they lose their group health coverage and do not have any other group health benefits plan available to them. Certain conditions must be met in order for this provision to apply, however. For example, individuals cannot decide not to enroll in their group's health insurance plan and then later change their minds when they need care. They must enroll when they have the opportunity to do so and not wait until they think they will need the coverage.

Specifically, HIPAA guarantees that, regardless of health status, individuals who have maintained continuous coverage and who then lose coverage under a group health plan may purchase coverage in the individual purchaser market. To be eligible for individual coverage under HIPAA, a person must

- have 18 or more months of aggregate creditable coverage (the most recent coverage must have come from a group health plan, government plan, or church plan or have been health insurance coverage linked to any such plan)
- be ineligible for group health coverage, Medicare, or Medicaid
- lack other health insurance coverage
- have not been terminated from his or her most recent prior coverage for nonpayment of premiums or fraud

- have elected and exhausted Consolidated Omnibus Reconciliation Act (COBRA) coverage or similar state-mandated
continuation coverage if he or she was eligible for it (CO-
BRA requires an employer to offer terminated employees
the opportunity to purchase continuation of health care coverage under the employer's medical plan for an 18-month
period [longer if the employees are disabled] or until eligible for another group health benefits plan).

Nothing in HIPAA controls the amount of premium that a
health insurer may charge for individual coverage. The act
does include specific details, however, about when enrollment
must occur and what circumstances must obtain for an individual to gain the protected access to health insurance the act
provides. The interested reader is referred to either the *Managed Health Care Handbook* or to the *HIPAA Compliance
Handbook.**

Medical Savings Accounts

Medical savings accounts are a way for individuals who do
not have group health insurance to pay for health care with
pre-tax dollars. Such an account requires the person to have
catastrophic insurance (i.e., health insurance with a very high
deductible and coinsurance) in order to be protected against
extremely high medical costs. Medical savings accounts were

---

*P.R. Kongstvedt, ed., *The Managed Health Care Handbook,* 4th ed.
Gaithersburg, MD: Aspen Publishers Inc., 2000.

HIPAA Compliance Handbook 2002, Gaithersburg, MD: Aspen Publishers, Inc., 2001.

initiated as a demonstration, and only a limited number were authorized. The program was recently extended, the accounts were renamed "Archer medical savings accounts," but their level of use remains low. Their ultimate usefulness is undetermined at this time.

Amendments to HIPAA

Three clinical conditions were addressed though amendments to the original act. The Newborns' and Mothers' Health Protection Act of 1996 mandates a minimum 48-hour length of stay for normal vaginal deliveries and a 96-hour length of stay for cesarean sections. The Mental Health Parity Act of 1996 requires that the aggregate lifetime dollar limits and annual dollar limits for mental health benefits and medical-surgical benefits be equal. Ironically, it does not actually require benefits plans to offer mental health benefits, nor does it require the same levels of co-payment or coinsurance if it does; it only requires the same lifetime and annual limits. The Women's Health and Cancer Rights Act of 1998 requires that group health plans, as well as health insurance that covers medical and surgical benefits for mastectomies, also provide coverage for (1) all stages of breast reconstruction, (2) surgery and reconstruction of the other breast to produce a symmetrical appearance, and (3) prostheses and physical complications of mastectomy.

Administrative Simplification

The section of HIPAA that concerns administrative simplification is currently the most important section of the law. The goal of this section is to reduce the administrative costs and burden in health care, standardize certain data elements, and protect the privacy of an individual's health information. All of the section's provisions are undergoing or have undergone a highly complex process of public commentary and final rule publication. The earliest any of these provisions would be applied is October 2002, and that date may be pushed forward. Four important issues that the administrative simplification section deals with are described below.

Transactions and Code Sets

The transactions in question are electronic transfers of data between providers and payers, among others, and the code sets are the definitions of the data. Prior to HIPAA, the transactions and code sets were not standardized to any great degree. The goal of the administrative simplification section of HIPAA is to create a single, uniform national standard for electronic transactions and thereby reduce errors, make the transactions easier and cheaper, and encourage their use by all parties. The transaction and code set provisions are the only HIPAA provisions that completely preempt state law.

The electronic transactions are defined using industry standards referred to as the ANSI ASCX12 Transactions, 40.10 release (American National Standards Institute, Accredited Standards Committee). They are as follows:

- **Health claims or equivalent encounter information.** This transaction is used by health care providers to submit health care claim billing information, encounter information, or both, to health plans.
- **Health claims attachments.** These attachments are used to transmit health care service information, such as subscriber,

patient, demographic, diagnosis, or treatment data, for the purposes of review, certification, or notification or for reporting the outcome of a health care services review.

- **Enrollment and disenrollment in a health plan.** This transaction is used to establish communication between the sponsor of health benefits and the health plan. It provides enrollment data, such as data on the subscriber and his or her dependents, as well as information on employers and health care providers. The "sponsor" is the backer of the coverage, benefit, or product. The sponsor can be an employer, union, government agency, association, or insurance company. The health plan is the entity that pays the claims, administers the insurance product or benefits, or both.

- **Eligibility for a health plan.** This transaction is used to inquire about the eligibility, coverage, or benefits associated with a benefits plan, an employer, a plan sponsor, a subscriber, or a dependent under a subscriber's policy. It also can be used to communicate information about or changes in eligibility, coverage, or benefits. Such information typically is sent by insurers, sponsors, and health plans, among other sources, and is sent to physicians, hospitals, third-party administrators, and government agencies, among other recipients.

- **Health care payment and remittance advice.** This transaction is used by a health plan to make a payment, send an explanation of benefits or remittance advice, or send both a payment and data to a health care provider.

- **Health plan premium payment.** This transaction is used by employers, employees, unions, associations, and other entities to make health plan premium payments to health insurers and keep track of these payments.

- **First report of injury.** This transaction is used to report information about an injury, illness, or incident to entities interested in the information for statistical, legal, claims, or risk management purposes.
- **Health claim status.** This transaction is used by health care providers and recipients of health care products or services to request from a health plan the status of a health care claim or encounter.
- **Referral certification and authorization.** This transaction is used to transmit health care service referral information between health care providers and health plans. It may also be used to obtain authorization for certain health care services from a health plan.

The code sets for these transactions are created by recognized standard-setting organizations and are already widely used. Not only does HIPAA require the use of these standard codes, it expressly prohibits the use of any other codes. In other words, neither an MCO nor a provider may use special codes that are not already part of these national code sets.

The HIPAA-mandated code sets are as follows:

- Volumes 1 and 2 of the *International Classification of Diseases,* ninth revision, clinical modification (*ICD-9-CM,* as updated and distributed by the U.S. Department of Health and Human Services [DHHS]), will be used for
  1. diseases
  2. injuries

3. impairments
4. other health problems and their manifestations
5. causes of all of the above
- Volume 3 of the ICD-9-CM will be used for the following procedures or actions provided to hospitals inpatients:
  1. prevention
  2. diagnosis
  3. treatment
  4. management
- The *National Drug Codes* (NDC, updated and distributed by DHHS) will be used for
  1. drugs
  2. biologics
- The Code on Dental Procedures and Nomenclature, or Common Dental Codes (CDT), will be used for dental services (updated and distributed by the American Dental Association).
- The *HCFA Common Procedure Coding System* (HCPCS, updated and distributed by DHHS) and *Current Procedural Terminology,* fourth edition (CPT-4, updated and distributed by the American Medical Association), will be used for
  1. physician services
  2. physical and occupational therapy services
  3. radiological procedures
  4. clinical laboratory tests
  5. other medical diagnostic procedures
  6. hearing and vision services
  7. transportation

National Identifiers

HIPAA mandates that uniform identifiers be used by all health plans, providers, and employers. None of the identifiers has been finalized at the time of this writing.

The identifier for an employer is the employer's tax identification number. No additional requirements are placed on employers.

The national identifier for a provider will replace all other identifiers in use except for the provider's tax identification number (which is only used for tax matters). Currently, a provider might have a multitude of different identifiers depending on whether the provider participates in an HMO, a PPO, Medicare, Medicaid, and so forth. The national identifier will replace all current identifiers so that the provider will have one and only one identifier for use in all circumstances.

The identifier for health plans has not yet been clearly defined. It is likely that each health benefits plan offered by an insurance company, MCO, or employer will have its own identifier.

Privacy

The privacy provisions of HIPAA are highly complex and are currently being modified. State provisions are allowed to be stricter than those of HIPAA but not less strict. The issue of privacy as dealt with by HIPAA encompasses the following subissues.

Consumer Control over Health Information. Patients have the right to understand and control how their health information is used. In particular, the following rules apply:

- Patients should be educated about privacy protections.
- Patients should have access to their medical records.
- Patient consent is required before information is released.
- Patient consent must be voluntary, not coerced.
- Patients should have recourse if their privacy protections are violated.

Limits on Medical Record Use and Release. With few exceptions, a patient's health information can be used for health care purposes only. In addition, in any circumstance, only the minimum necessary information should be disclosed (this rule does not apply to the transfer of medical records for the purpose of medical treatment). Further, routine disclosures require patient consent, and nonroutine disclosures require patient authorization.

Security of Personal Health Information. HIPAA establishes privacy safeguard standards that covered entities must meet but leaves detailed policies and procedures for meeting these standards to their discretion. Covered entities must

- adopt written privacy procedures
- take steps to ensure that their business associates protect the privacy of health information
- train employees and designate a privacy officer whose job is to ensure procedures are followed
- establish grievance processes that allow patients to inquire about the privacy of their records or file a complaint alleging an infringement of privacy

Accountability for Medical Records Use and Release. Penalties have been established for covered entities that misuse personal health information. Civil monetary penalties are $100 per incident and can accumulate up to $25,000 per person per year per standard. Federal criminal penalties can be as high as $250,000 and up to 10 years in prison for knowingly and improperly disclosing information or obtaining information under false pretenses.

Exceptions to Privacy Protection. DHHS has established rules that permit certain disclosures of health information without individual authorization. Unauthorized disclosures are allowed in the case of activities related to

- national defense and security
- public health
- judicial and administrative proceedings
- law enforcement (under limited conditions)

They are also sometimes allowed in circumstances in which the provision of care might otherwise be obstructed, such as a medical emergency, and for the purposes of health system oversight (including quality assurance), the identification of deceased persons, and the compilation of patient directories.

Security

The final rules for security have not yet been established, but a general understanding of what will be in those rules is possible. The rules will apply, for instance, to the following areas:

- administrative procedures
  1. authorization procedures for access to and modification of health care information
  2. policies and procedures regarding the use of passwords and security
  3. documented plans and procedures for dealing with emergencies
- physical safeguards
  1. safeguards restricting physical access to health information (e.g., locks on doors and secure information files)
  2. safeguards and security measures for the storage media used to maintain health information (e.g., the storage or shredding of paper records, the storage of data tapes, and the deletion of information from discarded computer hard drives)
- technical security services
  1. control of access to health information through the use of passwords, identifiers, and so forth
  2. prevention of access to health information by nonauthorized personnel through automatic logging off of computer terminals and so forth
  3. auditing of access to health information to determine who has seen it and for what reason
- technical security mechanisms
  1. secure computer transmission protocols for use on the network or the Internet
  2. digital signatures (although digital signatures are not actually required under HIPAA, if they are used, they must comply with certain rules)

SELF-INSURED EMPLOYERS AND THE EMPLOYEE RETIREMENT INCOME SECURITY ACT

The Employee Retirement Income Security Act of 1974 (ERISA) has had a direct impact on all health benefits plans and MCOs, especially self-funded plans. As discussed in Chapter 2, an employer has the option of assuming the risk for the medical costs associated with a health benefits plan rather than buying insurance to cover the risk. In a very real sense, a self-insured employer is acting as an insurance company. It is rare for a self-insured employer to administer its health plan, however. The more likely strategy is for it to contract with an insurance company or MCO to administer the plan.

Although the states regulate insurance, the federal government, under ERISA, regulates self-funded benefits plans and, to a limited degree, certain aspects of insured benefits plans. The degree of oversight and regulation is not comparable, however. ERISA, while it covers many administrative issues, does not address health issues to the same degree that state insurance departments do.

Even though it does not concern the business of insurance, ERISA does apply to aspects of employee benefits in general, including those in insured plans. Regarding these aspects, individual states are allowed to have requirements that are stricter but not less strict than those found in ERISA. These requirements primarily concern documentation (e.g., the requirement that a health benefits plan provide consumers with an intelligible description of the plan), although some of them cover the filing of information with the U.S. Department of Labor and the Internal Revenue Service.

Under ERISA, self-insured employers are not subject to any state laws regarding benefits or premiums or to any other oversight. Indeed, under the act, benefits and costs are hardly regulated at all. What little regulation there is addresses items such as

- exclusions for preexisting conditions
- waiting periods
- coverage of children (including adopted children and coverage of children through court order in divorce)
- pediatric vaccinations
- coverage for mental health services, maternity care, and mastectomies

ERISA does regulate how self-insured benefits plans deal with the payment of claims and appeals of denied claims. It specifies that a health plan must make a decision regarding an urgent care claim within 3 days, a preservice claim (i.e., a preauthorization for service) within 15 days, and a postservice claim within 30 days. One 15-day extension is allowed on pre- and postservice claims. For appeals, there is a 3-day limit on urgent care claims, a 30-day limit on preservice claims, and a 60-day limit on postservice claims. Patients have 180 days to file appeals.

ACCREDITATION OF MANAGED CARE ORGANIZATIONS

Accreditation is a form of oversight in which an outside organization reviews an MCO and determines if it meets certain criteria. If it meets those criteria (discussed below), it is considered accredited. The difference between accreditation and oversight by a government agency (e.g., a state insurance department) is that the accreditation organization is an independent, private, nonprofit entity. In essence, accreditation is a "seal of approval," and as such it is relied on by many employers, consumers, and even government agencies.

Accreditation agencies commonly look at an MCO's quality management program and its impact on operations, at utilization management and how it is carried out, at the MCO's treatment of members or consumers, and so forth. The criteria subject to review vary depending on the type of MCO and the accreditation agency performing the review. Below is a brief discussion of the commonly used accreditation agencies in managed care, followed by a description of the Health Plan Employer Data and Information Set (HEDIS) and some of the measures contained therein.

Accreditation Organizations

Three organizations have developed managed care oversight programs of note. Further, they approach their oversight role from different perspectives and specialize in different sectors of the market. The National Committee for Quality Assurance (NCQA), the Joint Commission on the Accreditation of Healthcare Organizations (Joint Commission), and the Utilization Review Accreditation Commission (URAC) all now accredit MCOs, and they all offer related accreditation or certification programs. In addition, NCQA has had a special impact on performance measurement in the world of managed care through its development of HEDIS, which is used by roughly 90 percent of all MCOs.

HMOs have been subjected to external accreditation review more than other types of MCOs. In fact, over 70 percent of HMOs have undergone review. NCQA is the dominant accreditation agency for HMOs, although URAC and the Joint Commission also have HMO programs. The accreditation process for HMOs is extensive. It looks at quality management, utilization management, wellness and prevention, the treatment of specific diseases and outcomes achieved, provider network composition and access, provider credentialing, financial performance, customer service and member satisfaction, grievance and appeal procedures, and other measures.

PPOs have not undergone accreditation review as commonly as HMOs, but that is changing. The main accrediting organization for PPOs is URAC, but again both NCQA and the Joint Commission have PPO programs. The accreditation process looks at many of the same topics as the process for HMOs, with some exceptions, including specific diseases. The process tends to be less detailed, which is consistent with the less intensive management of care provision characteristic of PPOs.

Free-standing utilization review organizations can also be accredited. Unsurprisingly, the focus of the accreditation reviews is on utilization management activities. URAC is the main accrediting organization for utilization review organizations.

Finally, provider organizations in managed care can be accredited, and the Joint Commission, which is virtually the sole accreditation organization for hospitals, is the main accreditation organization for providers.

HEDIS

HEDIS has become an industry standard for reporting data to employers and some government agencies. HEDIS, which was developed and is continually refined by NCQA, currently consists of about 60 measures that fall into seven broad categories:

1. *Effectiveness of Care.* Measures in this category underlie such frequently reported statistics as childhood immunization rates and mammography rates. These and other measures seek to establish whether the health plan is responding to the needs of those who are ill ("Does the health plan make me better when I am sick?") and also to the needs of those who are well ("Does the health plan keep me healthy when I am well?").

2. *Access/Availability of Care.* Measures in this category assess whether care is available to members when they need it. Accessibility is a precondition of high-quality care.

3. *Member Satisfaction.* The measures in this category provide important information about whether the health plan is able to satisfy the diverse needs of its members. Two surveys—one for adults, the other for exploring parents' impressions of the care their children receive—include questions related to key consumer issues, such as average office wait times, satisfaction with choice of provider, difficulty receiving care, and overall satisfaction.

4. *Use of Services.* How a health plan uses its resources is a sign of how efficiently care is managed. Measures look

at such factors as cesarean section rates, maternity length of stay, well-child visits, mental health utilization, and frequency of selected procedures.

5. *Cost of Care.* Used in conjunction with other measures, the measures in this category (rate trends, frequency of high-cost procedures) permit comparisons to be make between plans (in particular, the "value" of the services they deliver).

6. *Informed Health Care Choices.* Measures are currently being developed for this new category, which was added to encourage health plans to help members become active partners in their health care by providing them with enough information about treatment options to allow them to make informed choices.

7. *Health Plan Descriptive Information.* Although not technically measures, several general questions about the health plan are included because employers and consumers have found the resulting information useful when selecting among plans.

CONCLUSION

The managed care industry is heavily regulated and carefully scrutinized. MCOs, no matter what types of benefits plans they are selling and administering, are subject to federal and state laws and regulations. In addition, private nonprofit accreditation agencies are increasingly reviewing the operations of MCOs in order to assure consumers, employers, and government agencies that they are meeting quality and performance criteria.

Epilogue: Managed Health Care at the Millennium

THE ROLLERCOASTER THAT NEVER STOPS

The health care system in the United States has never settled into a prolonged state of peaceful equilibrium. Eighteenth-century medical practitioners were hampered by a lack of medical knowledge, and many treatments of the period caused more misery than the diseases they purported to cure. Health care in the nineteenth century can best be characterized as a free-for-all. Advances in medicine did occur, but their benefits were counterbalanced by the conferring of Doctor of Medicine degrees by a wide variety of medical schools, many of which barely provided an education and also promulgated strange and useless treatments. Furthermore, commerce entered medicine in a big way, leading to the proliferation of patent medicines, new "electrical cures," potions and nostrums guaranteed to cure any disease, and expensive spa treatments for the wealthy. Finally, during the twentieth century, the field of medical education was subjected to greater discipline, partly as a result of the Flexner Report, and science became a central part of medicine. Clinical advances began to accelerate—and have continued to accelerate at an increasing rate.

Until the middle of the twentieth century, medical care remained generally affordable, and physician fees accounted for most of the expense of care. Then technical advances and the growing use of hospitals led to higher costs, especially for those unfortunates who suffered from a serious illness or injury. At about the same time, insurance for catastrophic health care costs first appeared and a few prepaid medical care systems were inaugurated.

The health care system underwent a big change in 1965, when Congress passed legislation establishing Medicare and Medicaid. These two federal programs lit the fuse, and health care costs exploded off the launch pad. By the mid-1970s, health care cost inflation had hit third-party payers severely—employers, the federal government, and the state governments. Price controls, including prospective payments for hospitals and fee limits for physicians, were put into place to bring down the inflation rate. Health maintenance organizations (HMOs) were strongly supported by the federal government as a means of ensuring the affordability of care, and over time the private sector adopted managed care as the primary vehicle for keeping costs under control without reducing benefits to useless levels.

As indicated, the transformation of the health care system during the past 50 years has been extraordinary. Some of the changes have been beneficial, including improvements in many treatments and diagnostic tests. Others have not been, such as the rise in the number of the uninsured and the increase in the economic barriers to care. In short, whereas the "good old days" are a fantasy, the present state of medicine is far from ideal.

USING THE MAGIC EIGHT BALL: THE ANSWER IS HAZY—TRY AGAIN LATER

The past evolution of the health care system—from scientific advances to the adoption of managed care—has proven impossible to predict in detail. For example, in the early 1980s, many predicted that staff or group model HMOs would provide all health care by 1995; such HMOs have been dwindling in number and currently represent only a small percentage of total MCO enrollment. In the middle to late 1980s, many predicted that all health care would be paid for by capitation at the century's end; instead, capitation has spread only slowly and has actually been reduced or eliminated in some health plans. In the early to middle 1990s, many predicted that health care would be financed and delivered via large, vertically integrated megacorporations (known as integrated delivery systems [IDFs] or integrated delivery and financing systems [IDFSs]). Each of these massive corporations would own an insurance company or HMO, physician practices, hospitals, ancillary services, and whatever else it needed to deliver and finance health care. At this point, very few IDFSs are still standing, most of the survivors are struggling financially, and the IDFSs that attempted to hard-wire vertical integration suffered losses in the megamillions.

Correct predictions of the course of the health care system do occur (see, for example, J. Goldsmith, The U.S. Health Care System in the Year 2000, *JAMA* 256 (1986): 3371–3375.) However, "common wisdom" is commonly an overreaction to a trend rather than the result of a deep understanding of the complex forces at work. In fact, the health care system, especially the managed care sector, changes in a nonlinear manner—a hallmark of chaotic or complexly adapting systems. It is to chaotic systems that we must now turn.

THEY WERE RIGHT ALL ALONG: MANAGED HEALTH CARE *IS* IN CHAOS*

Chaotic or complexly adapting systems (CAS) theory is a branch of mathematics that was not possible until the advent of the supercomputer, which allows the modeling of vast quantities of data. The weather is one of the best examples of a complexly adapting system; other examples include the stock market, ecosystems, evolution, and the entire universe. Since the data are currently insufficient for a mathematical analysis of the health care system, it is not possible to prove that CAS theory as a whole applies to the health care system, but this system does exhibit several important attributes of complexly adapting systems, as described below.

---

*Thanks to Hindy Shaman and Jacquiline Lutz and special thanks to Jean Stanford for their invaluable contributions to the following discussion of chaos theory and health care markets. Planning in chaotic managed health care markets is also the subject P.R. Kongstvedt, H. Shama, J. Lutz, and J. Stanford, "The Managed Care Maze: Chaos Theory in Motion" (Washington, DC: Cap Gemini Ernst & Young, 1999), and P.R. Kongstvedt, H. Shama, J. Lutz, and J. Stanford, "Equilibrium at the Edge: Planning in Chaotic Managed Care Markets" (Washington, DC: Cap Gemini Ernst & Young, 1999). Electronic versions of these monographs may be downloaded by selecting "Research" from the Web site www.us.cgey.com/ind_serv/industry/health.

The object under study is a system that can be described and modeled. Though often characterized as a nonsystem, health care, because of the interrelationships that exist between the numerous components, undeniably is a system. Furthermore, although it is highly complex, we can model it to some degree. For example, actuaries can model the probabilities of certain diseases occurring in a large population, planners can anticipate the need for certain medical services in a community, and pharmaceutical manufacturers can project the demand for new drugs.

The system model is essentially nonlinear. Attempts have been made in the past to construct linear models of managed health care markets, but the resulting models, even if temporarily adopted, have ultimately proven inadequate. The best known was a model that depicted managed care market evolution as a series of stages. In the first stage, managed care is rare, whereas in the final stage, managed care is dominant, capitation is the predominant form of reimbursement, most provider systems are vertically integrated, utilization is low, and excesses in hospital beds and specialty physicians have vanished.

No actual market has all the traits supposedly characteristic of the final stage. For example, Minneapolis has a high level of managed care penetration and more vertical integration than most markets, but it has a low level of capitation. Southern California has a relatively high level of capitation (though global capitation has recently come into disfavor), but there are still excess hospital beds, and many of the organized provider groups have failed. Further, the number of specialty physicians has not decreased, neither in total nor as a percentage of all practicing physicians.

Vast, numerous forces affect the system. The future of the health care system is impossible to predict using a small set of variables. Simple supply and demand are confounded by third-party payment and the impact of each individual's medical condition (and the individual's resulting emotional state) on his or her choice of treatment. Geographic barriers or habits, languages spoken, ethnicity, transportation options, community health hazards, the unintended consequences of legislation, and so forth, interact in ways that are extremely difficult to comprehend. Further, many factors remain unrecognized, and thus we cannot take them or their effects into account in constructing our picture of the health care system.

Small changes in initial conditions may have large effects. For example, the personality of a health plan executive might lead him or her to decide to merge with another health plan and create a system that dominates the local market. Likewise, a health plan's purchase of real estate may affect its bond ratings and reduce its available capital, causing it to initiate a substantial increase in pricing. A financial officer's inexperience may cause him or her to use a faulty accrual methodology, leading to a massive downward restatement of earnings and a sharp increase in premium rates.

Initial conditions do not exist at a single point in the past. In the first example above, the executive's personality can be considered part of the initial conditions at the time he or she arrived to lead the health plan, but it can also be considered part of the initial conditions on the day he or she first met with the CEO of the competing health plan to talk about a merger. Furthermore, each and every event can be viewed as an initial condition for *something*. Finally, the effects of today's initial conditions will interact with the effects of past initial conditions and with the effects of future initial conditions, making the prediction of change a spectacularly complex task.

Feedback of current conditions affects subsequent results, usually with significant (but not random) variation. Feedback occurs, for example, when events external to a health plan lead to changes within the plan (or when one part of the plan affects another part). It includes information that comes into a health plan and influences internal actions or events. Feedback is often referred to as turbulence, especially when it influences events not just once but repeatedly (think of turbulent river rapids where the flow of water against rocks keeps the aquatic forces roiling).

Feedback can be seen in action when, for instance, health care trade magazines begin to tout a particular strategy and a large number of health care organizations immediately attempt to adopt it. The creation of physician-hospital organizations (PHOs) was once a top trend, and media stories supported it by extolling the virtues of these organizations. Consultants and law firms recognized market demand when they saw it and offered their services to help create PHOs. Most PHOs are now quiescent or have ceased to exist, although a few remain functional.

As another illustration, consider the actions of competitors within a given marketplace. Suppose a managed care plan decides to drop rates in an attempt to gain market share. The other plans would immediately respond with a rate decrease to remain competitive, and a rate war would ensue. The short-term benefits to employers of lowered rates would be negated by the rate increases that eventually would follow, not to mention the possibility that one of the plans would be too weak financially to subsidize rates for long and would go under.

HANDICAPPING THE FIELD: STRATIFYING FACTORS ACCORDING TO PREDICTABILITY

The term *chaos* (or even *complexly adapting system*) invokes feelings of helplessness—a fear of being unable to make predictions or choose right actions. While making predictions and acting appropriately in a chaotic environment are certainly more difficult than in a linear one, they are not impossible. Understanding the forces and factors that currently exist will allow an improved understanding of what the future *may* hold. The task, basically, is to counter entropy (defined here as the tendency for a system to become more chaotic unless energy is put into the system) by investing energy in strategy and management and applying an understanding of uncertainty and probability.

Predicting the future of managed care is a daunting task. If we demanded a high degree of certainty, we would be limited to making broad general statements, such as "Premium rates will go up by some amount next year." If we want more detailed predictions, we must accept that they will be fallible.

On the other hand, not all predictions are equally uncertain. Indeed, the factors that are currently having an influence on the health care system can be separated into those whose overall impact is relatively predictable and those whose overall impact is relatively unpredictable. By considering these factors and the effects they are likely to have, each of us may create our own vision of the future of managed care. The following sections contain lists of such factors as they exist in 2002.

Factors Having Relatively Predictable Consequences

Nonlegislative

- Increase in e-commerce by all parties
  1. Shift toward using electronic business processes and Web-enabled products and services
  2. Use of the Internet as a low cost means of automating the billions of transactions between health plans, providers, and consumers
  3. Increased use of electronic medical records
  4. Continued consolidation of e-Health businesses

- Slow and steady drift toward increased consumerism
  1. Increased enrollee demands on and expectations for health plans based on information from the Internet and the media
  2. Consumer desires for more and better information so consumers can participate in decisions about their health care
  3. More patients coming to doctor's appointments carrying material from the Internet (material not necessarily accurate or unbiased)
  4. More impatient patients

- Shifting demographics
  1. Increased life expectancy
     —Greater health needs later in life

—Proportionately smaller population base to fund health care costs

—Declining disability rates and higher expectations for good health

2. Increased ethnic diversity

3. Greater cost to society from rising number of uninsured people

- Continued consolidation of managed care plans and provider systems (but not to the point of creating national megacorporations)

- Perpetuation of market power at the regional and local levels

- Continued pressure of premium-cost compression in the market resulting in modest margins and periods of modest profits or even losses

- Increased market pressure to attain demonstrably higher levels of administrative and medical quality combined with unwillingness to pay significantly higher premium rates (i.e., high administrative and clinical quality is a requirement just to be in the market)

- Market pressure to develop broad medical networks

- Countervailing pressure to control costs

- Advances in medical technology in the areas of telemedicine, robotics, imaging, surgery, drug therapy, and gene therapy, among others

- Increasing ability to detect and treat asymptomatic diseases (e.g., hyperlipidemia and hypertension) with ever more sophisticated and costly drugs

- Increasing ability to detect and treat diseases early in their course (e.g., genetic diseases, diabetes, and precancerous states) with gene therapy and ever more sophisticated and costly drugs

Legislative

- Trend toward more regulation
  1. Mandatory second opinion programs and the like
  2. Market pressure to add consumer protections, whether actual danger exists or not
  3. Countervailing pressure from business community not to add to costs

- Consequences of the Health Insurance Portability and Accountability Act (HIPAA)
  1. Administrative simplification
  2. Increased privacy and security
  3. Limited portability of insurance

- Lack of an alternative to the private market for health insurance in the commercial sector (i.e., insufficient support for the replacement of private health insurance with a government-run single-payer health insurance system)

Factors Having Relatively Unpredictable Consequences

Nonlegislative

- Anti–managed care sentiment

- Ripple effects of failures of risk-bearing organizations

- Effect of the competition's strategies on health systems and health plans (an example of small causes with potentially large consequences)

- Effect of lawsuits (e.g., lawsuits against types of reimbursement, network restrictions, utilization management policies, and the like)

- High rates of evolution of provider structure and behavior

- High variation in provider structure and behavior in different geographic regions

- High variation in methods of compensating providers

- Possible employers' actions if costs increase above general inflation levels
  1. Use of purchasing marts
  2. Accelerated movement towards fixed contribution plans and movement away from defined benefit plans in which the employer pays any cost increases
  3. Movement back toward smaller, less costly networks

- Performance of U.S. economy
  1. Economic growth rate
  2. Unemployment rate

Legislative

- Unintended effects of federal legislation
  1. HIPAA
     —Cost to health plans and providers to remediate information systems (i.e., fix the actual computer code in order to make a system compliant)
     —Consequences of failure to comply with the act
     —Effect of standardization of transactions and identifiers on existing businesses that capitalize on the current lack of standardization
     —Increased use of the Internet for health care transactions and communication
       - Risk from e-vandals who attempt to damage the servers and Web sites of organizations
       - Risk from e-thieves who attempt to steal financial and medical information
       - Enormous increase in information available to consumers and physicians
  2. Balanced Budget Act of 1997
     —Decreased revenues to hospitals and diminished cost shifting
     —Change in the attractiveness of Medicare+ Choice risk plans as compared with existing health plans
     —Emergence of new types of risk-based health plans

- Erosion of the ERISA shield and increase in ability to file lawsuits against health plans and employers

- Decreasing ability of state governments to pay their portion of Medicaid

- Desire of state and federal governments to be out of the health insurance business

- Desire of state and federal governments to remain in the political business by creating unfunded mandates and compliance requirements

- Desire of CMS to increase Medicare managed care enrollment

- Countervailing desire of CMS to pay less for health care

- Use of risk-adjustors in calculating premiums paid by private employers and government agencies

- Federal legislation under debate or consideration
  1. The Patient's Bill of Rights
  2. Legislation that would revise the tax treatment of employee benefits plans

- Even-numbered year elections
  1. Presidential elections (every four years)
  2. Congressional elections (all representatives and one-third of senators every two years)

- Intended and unintended effects of state legislation and regulation
  1. State anti–managed care legislation
  2. State-specific mandates
  3. State regulatory interpretations

- Some new idea it is impossible to conjecture on (even though retrospectively it may seem obvious)

The above list of factors is not comprehensive—and could not be, because the health care system is a complexly adapting system. Furthermore, not all of them apply equally to any individual organization or situation. For example, a capital expenditure decision may not be influenced by a Patient's Bill of Rights but would be affected by the rise in e-commerce. Nonetheless, the exercise of stratifying factors according to their relative uncertainty must be undertaken when looking forward for purposes of predicting, planning, and acting.

DRIVING A NITROGLYCERIN TRUCK ON A FOGGY NIGHT: PREDICTING THE FUTURE

Henri-Georges Clouzot's wonderful 1953 movie *The Wages of Fear* is about four criminals who drive trucks containing extremely unstable nitroglycerin across rugged terrain in South America. Making predictions about managed care may not be as physically dangerous, but it does have an equally high probability of blowing up in one's face.

Most people and most organizations seek stability. There is only so much change that can be absorbed before feelings of exhaustion set in and the desire to slow down or stop change becomes paramount. Stability, though, is the one thing that has been lacking in the health care system and will continued to be lacking in the foreseeable future. In a chaotic market, it is dangerous to predict the future based on only a few variables or market attributes.

It is the sincere hope of this author that this book has provided the reader with a solid understanding of the basic elements of managed health care—an understanding of what it actually is and an understanding of how the various parts work. As for predicting the future, you are now more equipped than before to make your own predictions. As for me, I plan to shake the Magic Eight Ball.

—PRK
February, 2002

Glossary

24/7 Slang for "available 24 hours a day, 7 days a week."

accrete The term used by CMS to refer to the process of adding new Medicare enrollees to a plan. *See also* **delete.**

accrual The amount of money set aside by a plan to cover expenses. The plan's best estimate of what its expenses are, the accrual is based on a combination of data from the authorization system, the claims system, lag studies, and the plan's prior history.

ACS (Administrative Contract Services) contract *See* **administrative services only (ASO) contract.**

actuarial assumptions The assumptions that an actuary uses in calculating the expected costs and revenues of a plan. Examples include the utilization rate, age, and sex mix of enrollees and the cost for medical services.

adjusted average per capita cost (AAPCC) Best estimate from CMS of the amount of money it costs to care for Medicare recipients under fee-for-service Medicare in a given area. The measure is made up of 142 different rate cells; 140 of them are factored for age, sex, Medicaid eligibility, institutional status, working aged (i.e., those individuals who qualify for Medicare by virtue of their age, but who work full time and are therefore covered primarily by their commercial health plan), and whether a person has both Part A and Part B of Medicare. The 2 remaining cells are for individuals with end-stage renal disease.

adjusted community rate (ACR) Used by HMOs and CMPs [Competitive Medical Plan (a term used by CMS to designate a non-federally qualified HMO that qualifies for Medicare+Choice)] with Medicare risk contracts to determine the premium to charge for providing exactly the Medicare-covered benefits to a group account adjusted to allow for the greater intensity and frequency of utilization by Medicare recipients. The ACR, which includes the normal profit of a for-profit HMO or CMP, may be equal to or lower than the **average payment rate** (see below) but can never exceed it.

administrative services only (ASO) contract A contract between an insurance company and a self-funded plan according to which the insurance company performs administrative services only and does not assume any risk. The services usually include claims processing but may include other services as well, such as actuarial analysis, utilization review, and so forth. *See also* **Employee Retirement Income Security Act.**

adverse selection The problem of attracting members who are sicker than the general population (specifically, members who are sicker than was anticipated when the budget for medical costs was developed).

AFDC *See* **Temporary Assistance to Needy Families.**

ALOS *See* **length of stay.**

Amara's Law The tendency, when confronted with significant change, to overreact in the short term and underreact in the long term. The author gratefully acknowledges Greg Lippe as the source of this highly useful aphorism.

ambulatory care groups (ACGs) Used to categorize outpatient episodes. These 51 groups are mutually exclusive and are based on resource use over time and modified by principle diagnosis, age, and sex. *See also* **ambulatory diagnostic groups; ambulatory patient classifications; ambulatory patient groups.**

ambulatory diagnostic groups (ADGs) Used to categorize outpatient episodes. There are 34 possible ADGs. *See also* **ambulatory care groups; ambulatory patient groups.**

ambulatory patient classifications (APCs) Used by CMS for implementing the prospective payment system for ambulatory procedures. Like other classification systems, the APC system clusters many different ambulatory procedure codes into categories for purposes of payment.

ambulatory patient groups (APGs) APGs were developed by 3M Health Information Systems for the Health Care Financing Administration (now CMS), which has still not implemented them (though some commercial MCOs have). APGs are to outpatient procedures what DRGs are to inpatient days. APGs provide for a fixed reimbursement to an institution for outpatient procedures or visits and incorporate patient data and data on the reason for the visit. APGs prevent unbundling of ancillary services. *See also* **ambulatory care groups; ambulatory diagnostic groups; ambulatory patient classifications.**

American Accreditation Healthcare Commission (AAHC) *See* **Utilization Review Accreditation Commission.**

American Association of Health Plans (AAHP) AAHP is the primary trade organization for managed care organizations. It focuses on legislation, lobbying, education, certification of training in managed care operations, and representing the managed care industry to the public. It was created in 1995 through the merger of the Group Health Association of America (GHAA) and the American Managed Care and Review Association (AMCRA), two predecessor organizations that represented slightly different health plan constituencies.

American National Standards Institute (ANSI) ANSI develops and maintains standards for electronic data interchange. The Health Insurance Portability and Accountability Act mandates the use of ANSI ASCX12N standards for electronic transactions in the health care system.

any willing provider (AWP) An "any willing provider" law requires an MCO to accept any provider willing to meet the terms and conditions in the MCO's contract whether the MCO wants or needs that provider. This type of state law is considered to be an expensive variety of anti–managed care legislation.

assignment of benefits The payment of medical benefits directly to a provider of care rather than to a member. Generally requires either a contract between the health plan and the provider or a written release from the subscriber to the provider allowing the provider to bill the health plan.

automated clearinghouse (ACH) A company that accepts claims or other transactions from providers, reformats them into standards acceptable to each payer, and electronically transmits them to the payer. Prior to the Health Insurance Portability and Accountability Act, there were no functional standards in transaction definitions or data fields (there were standard definitions but the payers continued to use their own). With the advent of the act, the need for translation into multiple proprietary formats diminished considerably, but a company that will convert paper forms into electronic transactions still has considerable value for small provider groups.

average payment rate (APR) The amount of money that the CMS could conceivably pay an HMO or CMP for services provided to Medicare recipients under a risk contract. The amount is derived from the adjusted average per capita cost for the service area adjusted for the enrollment characteristics that the plan would expect to have. The payment to the plan (the adjusted community rate) can never be higher than the APR but it may be less.

average wholesale price (AWP) Commonly used in pharmacy contracting. The AWP is generally determined through reference to a common source of information such as a nationally published price or cost list.

balance billing The practice of a provider billing a patient for all charges not paid for by the insurance plan even if those charges are above the plan's usual, customary, or reasonable charges or the services are considered medically unnecessary. Managed care plans and service plans generally prohibit providers from balance billing except for allowed co-pays, coinsurance, and deductibles. Such prohibition against balance billing may even apply to situations where the plan fails to pay at all (e.g., because of bankruptcy).

Balanced Budget Act of 1997 A sweeping piece of legislation that created the Medicare+Choice program as well as demonstration medical savings accounts.

capitation A set amount of money received or paid out. The capitation rate for a plan is based on plan's membership rather than on services delivered and usually is expressed in units of per member per month (PMPM). The capitation rate for an enrolled member may be affected by factors such as the member's age and sex.

carve out Used to refer to medical services "carved out" of the basic set of services. In the case of plan benefits, a set of benefits might be contracted for separately. For example, mental health or substance abuse services may be separated from basic medical-surgical services. A set of services may also be carved out of the basic capitation fee. For example, the capitation fee may cover cardiac care, but case rates might apply to cardiac surgery.

case management A method of managing the provision of health care to members with high-cost medical conditions. The goal is to coordinate the care so as to improve continuity and quality of care as well as lower costs. Case management is generally a dedicated function of the utilization management department. The Certification of Insurance Rehabilitation Specialists Commission defines case management as "a collaborative process which assesses, plans, implements, coordinates, monitors, and evaluates the options and services required to meet an individual's health needs, using communication and available resources to promote quality, cost-effective outcomes." According to the definition, case management "occurs across a continuum of care, addressing ongoing individual needs" rather than being restricted to a single practice setting. When focused solely on high-cost inpatient cases, it may be referred to as *large case management* or *catastrophic case management*.

case mix The mix of the diseases and the severity of the cases under treatment by a provider.

Centers for Medicare & Medicaid Services (CMS) The federal agency responsible for financing and overseeing Medicare and Medicaid services. CMS is part of the U.S. Department of Health and Human Services and was formerly known as the **Health Care Financing Administration** (HCFA).

certificate of authority (COA) The state-issued operating license for an HMO.

certificate of need (CON) The requirement that a health care organization obtain permission from an oversight agency before making changes. This requirement generally applies only to facilities or facility-based services.

CHAMPUS (Civilian Health and Medical Program of the Uniformed Services) Federal program that provides health care coverage to families of military personnel, military retirees, certain spouses and dependents of such personnel, and certain others. Currently provided via the TRICARE program. *See also* **Military Health System; TRICARE**.

Children's Health Insurance Program (CHIP) Also referred to as *State Children's Health Insurance Program (SCHIP)*. A program created by the federal government to provide a "safety net" and preventive-care level of health coverage for children. The program is funded through a combination of federal and state funds and administered by the states in conformance with federal requirements.

clean claim A claim for which there are no inherent reasons not to pay. Clean claims can be contrasted with pended claims (claims placed on hold), which include claims containing mistakes or incomplete data (e.g., an incorrectly entered provider identifier), claims possibly subject to other party liability, duplicate claims, claims in which the fees charged do not match the procedures done, and claims in which the procedures do not match the diagnoses.

closed-panel MCO An MCO that contracts with physicians on an exclusive basis for services and does not allow those physicians to see patients for another MCO. Examples include staff and group model HMOs, but a large private medical group that contracts with an HMO could be considered a closed panel MCO.

coinsurance Refers to an insurance provision that limits the amount of coverage for services to a certain percentage, commonly 80 percent. The rest of the cost is paid by the member out of pocket.

commission The money paid to a sales representative, broker, or other type of sales agent for selling the health plan. It may be a flat amount of money or a percentage of the premium.

community rating Rating methodology required of federally qualified HMOs, HMOs under the laws of many states, and indemnity plans under certain circumstances. If an HMO uses community rating, it basically charges the same amount to all members in the plan, although it can vary the rate somewhat by factoring in age, sex, mix (average contract size), and industry factors (not all factors are necessarily allowed under state laws, however). Rating in which such factors influence the amount charged is referred to as *community rating by class* and *adjusted community rating. See also* **experience rating.**

complementary and alternative medicine (CAM) Treatment modalities other than traditional allopathic medicine. Examples include acupuncture, chiropractic medicine, homeopathy, and various forms of "natural healing."

concurrent review Utilization management that takes place during the provision of services. It is applied to inpatient hospital stays almost exclusively.

Consolidated Omnibus Reconciliation Act (COBRA) Act requiring an employer to offer terminated employees the opportunity to purchase continuation of health care coverage under the group's medical plan (*see also* **conversion**). The act also makes it easier for a Medicare recipient to disenroll from an HMO or CMP with a Medicare risk contract.

Consumer Assessment of Health Plan Survey (CAHPS) Federal initiative intended to develop a set of satisfaction surveys built on a core of standardized items. The core can be supplemented by additional targeted elements to construct surveys adaptable to different subpopulations and suitable for making cross-group comparisons. Special Medicaid survey modules have been developed that accommodate educational, linguistic, and cultural differences in the Medicaid population.

contract year The 12-month period that a contract for services is in force. The contract year is not necessarily tied to a calendar year.

conversion The conversion of coverage under a group master contract to coverage under an individual contract. The chance to convert is offered to subscribers who lose their group coverage (e.g., through job loss or death of a working spouse) and who are ineligible for coverage under another group contract. *See also* **Consolidated Omnibus Reconciliation Act**.

coordination of benefits (COB) An agreement that uses language developed by the National Association of Insurance Commissioners and prevents double payment for services when a subscriber has coverage from two or more sources. For example, a husband may have Blue Cross Blue Shield through work, and the wife may be enrolled in an HMO through her place of employment. The agreement defines which organization has primary responsibility for payment and which has secondary responsibility. The primary and secondary payment obligations of the two organizations are determined by the Order of Benefits Determination Rules contained in the National Association of Insurance Commissioners (NAIC) Model COB Regulation as interpreted and adopted by the various states.

co-payment The amount that a member must pay out of pocket for medical services. It is usually a fixed amount, and in many HMOs it is only ten dollars.

corporate compliance Health plan or provider function charged with ensuring compliance with Medicare rules and regulations. These regulations also require the existence of a corporate compliance officer (CCO).

Corporate Practice of Medicine Acts or Statutes State laws that prohibit a physician from working for a corporation; in other words, a physician can only work for him or herself, or another physician. Put another way, a corporation cannot practice medicine. Often created through the effort on the part of certain members of the medical community to prevent physicians from working directly for managed care plans or hospitals.

cost sharing Payment by a member of some portion of the cost of services. Usual forms of cost sharing include deductibles, coinsurance, and co-payments.

cost shifting Raising the prices charged to other payers to cover the cost of providing services where the reimbursement received does not fully cover the cost.

credentialing Obtaining and reviewing the documentation of professional providers. Such documentation includes licenses, certifications, insurance, evidence of malpractice insurance, and malpractice history. Credentialing generally includes both reviewing information provided by a provider as well as verifying that the information is correct and complete. The term *credentialing* also refers to obtaining hospital privileges and other privileges to practice medicine.

Current Procedural Terminology, 4th edition (CPT-4) A set of five-digit codes that apply to medical services delivered. The codes are frequently used for billing purposes by professionals. *See also* **HCFA Common Procedural Coding System**.

date of service The date that medical services were rendered. The date of service is usually different from the date a claim is submitted.

days per thousand A standard unit for measuring the utilization of the hospital or other institutional care. The days per thousand are the number of hospital days used annually for each thousand covered lives.

death spiral The vicious spiral of high premium rates and adverse selection that can affect an insurance company or health plan in a free-choice environment. For example, one plan in a market, such as an indemnity plan competing with managed care plans, might have to raise its premium rates to cover costs, thus driving away some healthy members, which in turn causes an additional hike in rates to cover the costs of the generally less healthy members who remain, which drives away more of the healthy members, and so on, until the only members left are those who cannot change plans because of provider loyalty or benefits restrictions (e.g., preexisting conditions) and whose medical costs are so high that they far exceed any possible premium revenue. The name comes from the fact that the losses from underwriting mount faster than the gains from the premium payments, leading to the eventual termination of coverage and leaving the carrier in a permanent loss position.

deductible That portion of a subscriber's (or member's) health care expenses that must be paid out of pocket before the insurance coverage applies (usually $100 to $300). Deductibles are common in insurance plans and PPOs, uncommon in HMOs, and they may apply only to the out-of-network portion of a point-of-service plan or only to one portion of the plan coverage (e.g., just to pharmacy services).

defined benefit A benefit provided by an employer or government agency to all employees in which the design of the benefits plan (i.e, the type of coverage) has been selected by the employer, rather than forcing each employee to find and purchase health insurance on their own. Some degree of flexibility in selecting levels of coverage is common, but only within a limited range of choices offered by the employer. In other words, the employees know what types of insurance or managed health care plans are offered and what the benefits are under each, and the employer's contribution to the meeting the cost of the coverage is a function of how expensive the coverage is. This is the most common form of employee health insurance benefit.

defined contribution A fixed amount of money provided by an employer to employees for use in purchasing health insurance but without any requirement that the employees use it to enroll in health plans chosen by the employer.

delete The term used by CMS to refer to the process of removing Medicare enrollees from a plan. *See also* **accrete.**

dependent A member who has health care coverage in virtue of a family relationship. For example, the spouse and children of an individual with health insurance through work typically also have coverage under the contract.

DHHS See **U.S. Department of Health and Human Services.**

diagnosis-related groups (DRGs) A statistical system for classifying inpatient stays for purposes of payment. DRGs may be primary or secondary, and an outlier classification also exists. DRGs are used by CMS to pay hospitals for Medicare enrollees, and they are also used by a few states for all payers and by many private (usually non-HMO) health plans for contracting purposes.

Diagnostic and Statistical Manual of Mental Disorders, 4th Edition (DSM IV) A manual containing a diagnostic coding system for mental and substance abuse disorders. This manual is far different from the **International Classification of Diseases, Ninth Revision, Clinical Modification** (see below).

direct access Access to specialists without having to go through a primary care provider "gatekeeper." In an HMO that uses the direct access model, a member may self-refer to a specialist rather than having to seek an authorization. In such HMOs, the co-payment for care received from a specialist is usually much higher than the co-pay for care received from a primary care provider.

direct contracting Contracting that is between a provider or integrated health care delivery system and an employer and is unmediated by an insurance company or managed care organization. Direct contracting is a superficially attractive option that occasionally works when the employer is large enough. It is not to be confused with the **direct contract model** (see below).

direct contract model A model in which a managed care health plan contracts directly with private practice physicians in the community rather than through an intermediary such as an independent practice association or a medical group. Open-panel HMOs commonly use this model.

discharge planning That part of utilization management that is concerned with arranging for care or medical needs to facilitate discharge from the hospital.

disease management The process of intensively managing a particular disease. Disease management differs from large case management in that it goes well beyond managing the care of a patient during a single hospital stay or treating an acute exacerbation of a condition. Instead, it encompasses all settings of care and places a heavy emphasis on prevention and maintenance. Disease management is commonly used for a defined set of diseases.

disenrollment Termination of coverage. Disenrollment may be voluntary, such as when a member simply wants out, or involuntary, such as when a member leaves the plan because of a change of jobs. Rarely, a plan will terminate a member's coverage against the member's will. Such termination is usually only allowed (under state and federal laws) for gross offenses such as fraud, abuse, nonpayment of premium or co-payments, or a demonstrated inability to comply with recommended treatment plans.

dispense as written (DAW) The instruction from a physician to a pharmacist to dispense a brand-name pharmaceutical rather than a generic substitution.

DOL *See* **U.S. Department of Labor.**

drug utilization review (DUR) The tools and techniques to manage utilization of drugs. Similar in concept to utilization management in general, but focusing strictly on pharmacy benefit use and cost.

duplicate claim A claim is submitted a second time, usually because payment has not been received quickly. Duplicate claims can lead to duplicate payments and the entry of incorrect data in the claims file.

durable medical equipment (DME) Medical equipment that is not disposable (i.e., is used repeatedly). Examples include wheelchairs, home hospital beds, and so forth. Durable medical equipment is an area of increasing expense, particularly in conjunction with case management.

e-commerce The use of electronic communications to conduct business. By convention, e-commerce applies to the use of the Internet for business transactions. Also by convention, the "e" is almost always lowercase. e e cummings would approve.

effective date The day that health plan coverage goes into effect or is modified.

electronic data interchange (EDI) The exchange of data through electronic means rather than by using paper or the telephone. Prior to the rise of the Internet, the term applied primarily to direct electronic communications via proprietary means, but it now encompasses electronic data exchange via the Internet as well. The term *e-commerce,* however, is used most often for Internet-based electronic data exchange.

electronic funds transfer (EFT) Transfer of funds electronically instead through use of a paper check.

eligibility Meeting the qualifications for coverage under a plan. An individual eligible for coverage can become ineligible, as when a dependent child reaches a certain age and is no longer eligible for coverage under his or her parent's health plan.

emergency department (ED) A department in a hospital or other institutional facility that is focused on caring for acutely ill or injured patients. In earlier times, these patients were treated in a special room or set of rooms, hence the older designation *emergency room* (or *ER*). These days, at least in busy urban and suburban hospitals, where volume is high, emergency treatment is provided by an entire department staffed by physicians specially trained and certified in emergency care.

Emergency Medical Treatment and Active Labor Act (EMTALA) An act passed in 1986 that dictates that all patients presenting to a hospital emergency department must have a medical screening exam performed by qualified personnel, usually an emergency physician. The medical screening exam cannot be delayed for insurance reasons, either to obtain insurance information or to obtain preauthorization for examination. The act states, "An emergency medical condition means a medical condition manifested by acute symptoms of sufficient severity (including severe pain) that the absence of immediate medical attention could reasonably be expected to result in: a) placing the patient's health in serious jeopardy; b) serious impairment to bodily functions; or c) serious dysfunction of any bodily organ or part."

emergency room (ER) *See* **emergency department.**

employee assistance program (EAP) A program that a company puts into effect for its employees to provide them with help in dealing with personal problems, such as alcohol or drug abuse and mental health and stress-related problems.

Employee Retirement Income Security Act (ERISA) Act containing numerous provisions a managed care organization must be familiar with. One provision allows self-funded plans to avoid paying premium taxes, complying with state mandates regarding benefits, or otherwise complying with state laws and regulations regarding insurance, even when insurance companies and managed care plans that stand risk for medical costs must do so. Another provision requires that plans and insurance companies provide an explanation of benefits (EOB) statement to a member or covered insured in the event of a denial of a claim; the statement must explain why the claim was denied and inform the individual of his or her rights of appeal.

encounter An ambulatory visit by a member to a provider. The term applies primarily to physician office visits but may encompass other types of encounters as well. In fee-for-service plans, an encounter also generates a claim. In capitated plans, an encounter is still a visit, but no claim is generated.

enrollee An individual enrolled in a managed health care plan. The term usually applies to the subscriber (i.e., the person who has coverage in the first place) rather than to the subscriber's dependents, but it is not always used that precisely.

evidence of coverage (EOC) Also known as a *certificate of benefits*. The EOC is a document that describes the health care benefits covered by a health plan, explains how the coverage works, and provides authentication that the member does in fact have health insurance.

evidence of insurability A form that documents eligibility for health plan coverage for individuals not enrolling during an open enrollment period. For example, if an employee wants to change health plans in the middle of a contract year, the new health plan may require evidence of insurability (often both a questionnaire and a medical exam) to ensure that it will not be accepting adverse risk.

exclusive provider organization (EPO) An organization similar to an HMO in that it often uses primary physicians as gatekeepers, often capitates providers, has a limited provider panel, and uses an authorization system, among other points of likeness. It is referred to as exclusive because the member must remain within the network to receive benefits. The main difference between EPOs and HMOs is that the former are generally regulated under insurance statutes instead of HMO regulations. Many states disallow EPOs based on the premise that they are really HMOs.

expedited review A special form of external review used in an appeals program in cases where the medical services under dispute are of an urgent nature. As an example, if a patient requests a transplant that the MCO's medical policy classifies as experimental, the review of the MCO's denial of payment would be expedited so that the patient could undergo the transplant operation in a timely fashion in the eventuality the denial was overturned.

experience rating Setting premium rates for a group based on the group's historical health care costs.

explanation of benefits (EOB) statement A statement mailed to a member or covered insured explaining how and why a claim was paid or why it was not paid. The Medicare version is called an *EOMB* (*see also* **Employee Retirement Income Security Act**).

extracontractual benefits Health care benefits beyond what the member's policy covers. These benefits are provided by a plan in order to reduce utilization. For example, a plan may not provide coverage for a hospital bed at home but may provide such a bed nonetheless if it is more cost effective than repeatedly admitting the member to the hospital.

Federal Employee Health Benefits Program (FEHBP) The program that provides health benefits to federal employees. *See* **Office of Personnel Management.**

federal qualification A status achieved by HMOs and CMPs that meet federal standards regarding benefits, financial solvency, rating methods, marketing, member services, health care delivery systems, and other standards. An HMO or CMP must apply for federal qualification and be examined by the Office of Managed Care (the examination process includes an on-site review). Federal qualification does place some restrictions on how a plan operates but also expedites its entry into the Medicare and Federal Employee Health Benefits Program markets. Federal qualification is voluntary and is not required for entry into these markets.

fee-for-service (FFS) Used to describe a reimbursement system in which a provider bills a health plan or a patient for services actually provided. Fee-for-service reimbursement contrasts with capitation, where providers receive regular payments whether services are provided or not.

fee schedule Also called *fee maximums* or *fee allowance schedule.* A fee schedule is a list of the maximum fees that a health plan will pay for services.

flexible benefits plan A benefits plan in which employees are allowed to choose from a variety of benefits up to a certain total amount. In this type of plan, an employee can tailor the benefits package to his or her particular needs. For example, the employee might choose health coverage, life insurance, child care, and so forth.

formulary A list of drugs that a physician may prescribe (e.g., a list of drugs approved for use within a health care setting). The physician is requested or required to use only formulary drugs unless there is a valid medical reason to use a nonformulary drug.

foundation A type of nonprofit integrated health care delivery system. The foundation model is often implemented in response to tax laws that affect nonprofit hospitals or in response to state laws prohibiting the corporate practice of medicine (*see* **Corporate Practice of Medicine Acts or Statutes**). As an example, a foundation might be formed to purchase the tangible and intangible assets of a group practice, at which point the physicians would form a medical group to contract with the foundation on an exclusive basis for services to patients seen through the foundation.

full professional risk capitation Capitation received by a physician group for all medical services, not just for the services the group physicians themselves provide. The group is responsible for subcapitating or otherwise reimbursing other physicians for services provided to their members. Full professional risk capitation, unlike **global capitation** (see below), does not cover institutional services.

full-time equivalent (FTE) The equivalent of one full-time employee. For example, two half-time employees make up one FTE.

gag clause A clause in a provider contract that prevents a physician from telling a patient about certain available clinical treatment options. This clause is much like the Sasquatch—big, hairy, and scary but hard to find. The federal government conducted a review of managed care physician contracts and was unable to find any examples. Gag clauses have been banned by many states, and federal legislation is likely as well (it is at least *politically* useful to ban what does not exist anyway). Most or all contracts between MCOs and physicians do contain clauses that prohibit the physician from revealing business secrets such as reimbursement schedules, but this is a different matter. In the past, a contract might include provisions requiring a physician to contact the MCO before initiating a treatment option, and such provisions may have been interpreted or treated as gag clauses, but the majority of contracts actually require physicians to actively discuss options with their patients.

gatekeeper A primary care provider who has the authority to permit or deny access to other providers. In the primary care case management model, all care from providers other than the primary care provider must be authorized by the primary care provider before care is rendered, except in an emergency. Almost all HMOs use primary care providers as gatekeepers.

generic drug A drug that is equivalent to a brand-name drug but usually less expensive. Most MCOs that provide drug benefits cover generic drugs. Indeed, if a generic drug could be used to fill a prescription, an MCO may require a member who wants the brand-name drug to pay the difference in cost or pay a higher co-pay.

global capitation Capitation received by an organization for all services, including institutional, professional, and ancillary medical services.

group Members receiving health plan coverage at a single company.

group model HMO An HMO that contracts with a medical group for the provision of health care services. The relationship between the HMO and the medical group is generally very close, although there are wide variations in the degree of independence between the two. A group model HMO is a type of closed-panel health plan.

group practice The American Medical Association defines a group practice as three or more physicians who deliver patient care, make joint use of equipment and personnel, and divide income by a prearranged formula.

group practice without walls (GPWW) A group practice in which the members of the group come together legally, but continue to practice in private offices scattered throughout the service area. Sometimes called a *clinic without walls (CWW)*.

HCFA-1500 A claims form used by professionals to bill for services. Required by Medicare and generally used by private insurance companies and managed care plans for paper claims.

HCFA Common Procedural Coding System (HCPCS) HCPCS is a nationally defined set of codes used by Medicare to describe services, and has provisions for local use of certain codes; however, under HIPAA, all use of local codes is eliminated, and at the time of publication, it is not entirely clear which of the national HCPCS codes will remain in use. HCPCS includes CPT codes but also has codes not included in CPT, such as codes for durable medical equipment and ambulance services. Note that HCFA is now known as CMS.

health care You think you know what *health care* means? Well, maybe, maybe not. The term is generally used to refer to the services provided by health care professionals, and discussions of care management invariably use the term thusly. However, in a broader sense, *health care* encompasses services from nontraditional providers and, more importantly, self-administered care (the type of health care people mostly receive). When individuals employ the broad sense of *health care,* they frequently employ *medical care* to refer to the services provided by professionals.

Health Care Financing Administration (HCFA) The federal agency that oversees all aspects of health financing for Medicare and also oversees the Office of Managed Care. HCFA is part of the U.S. Department of Health and Human Services and is now known as the **Centers for Medicare & Medicaid Services** (CMS).

Health Insurance Association of America (HIAA) A trade organization that represents health insurance companies, whether or not those companies are managed health care organizations. The primary focus of HIAA has been on legislative and lobbying activities, though it has expanded its scope somewhat to include operational issues.

Health Insurance Portability and Accountability Act (HIPAA) An act passed in 1996 that created a set of requirements that allow for insurance portability (i.e., the ability of people to keep their health insurance even if they lose their eligibility for group health insurance). The act also guarantees the issuing of all health insurance products to small groups (but only if they have met requirements for prior continuous coverage) and mental health parity (i.e., the dollar limits on mental health coverage cannot be less than that those on medical coverage). It is silent, however, on the issues of differential visit limitations, differential coinsurance requirements, and restrictions on networks. The act also contains significant provisions regarding administrative simplification and privacy standards.

health maintenance organization (HMO) Originally, an organization that provided health care to voluntarily enrolled members who paid a capitation rate. With the increase in self-insured employers and financial arrangements that do not rely on prepayment, that definition is no longer accurate. The new definition must encompass licensed health plans (i.e., licensed as HMOs) that place at least some of the providers at risk for medical expenses and health plans that utilize designated providers (usually primary care physicians) as gatekeepers (although there are some HMOs that do not). Many in the field have given up and now use *managed care organization* to avoid the difficult task of fashioning a definition for the term.

Health Plan Employer Data Information Set (HEDIS) An ever-evolving set of data-reporting standards. Developed by the National Committee on Quality Assurance with considerable input from the employer community and the managed care community, HEDIS is designed to provide some standardization in the reporting of financial, utilization, membership, and clinical data so that employers and others can compare the performance of different plans.

health risk appraisals Instruments designed to elicit or compile information about the health risk of any given individual. Initially these instruments were fairly uniform, but recently they have become quite specialized and are targeted toward particular populations with distinctive risk profiles (Medicare enrollees, Medicaid recipients, the underserved population, the commercial population, and so forth).

HHS *See* **U.S. Department of Health and Human Services.**

hospitalist A physician who concentrates solely on hospitalized patients. In an MCO or a medical group, physicians may specialize in hospital care or hospital duties may be assigned on a rotating basis. The hospitalist model allows the other physicians to concentrate on outpatient care.

incurred but not reported (IBNR) Medical expenses that a plan has incurred but knows nothing about yet—medical expenses the authorization system has not captured or for which claims have not yet hit the door. Unexpectedly high IBNRs have torpedoed more managed care plans than any other cause.

independent practice association (IPA) An organization that has a contract with a managed care plan to deliver services in return for a single capitation rate. The IPA in turn contracts with individual providers to provide the services either on a capitation basis or on a fee-for-service basis. The typical IPA encompasses all specialties, but an IPA can be solely for primary care or for a single specialty. An IPA can also be the physician part of a **physician-hospital organization** (see below).

integrated delivery system (IDS) Also called an *integrated health care delivery system, integrated delivery network, integrated delivery and financing system,* and *integrated delivery and financing network.* An IDS is an organized system of health care providers that offers a broad range of health care services. Although not precisely definable, an IDS should be able to access the market on a broad basis, optimize cost and clinical outcomes, accept and manage a full range of financial arrangements for providing a set of defined benefits to a defined population, align the financial incentives of the participants (including physicians), and operate under a cohesive management structure. *See also* **foundation; independent practice association; management service organization; physician-hospital organization; staff model HMO.**

International Classification of Diseases, Ninth Revision, Clinical Modification (ICD-9-CM) A classification of disease by diagnosis codified into 6-digit numbers. The tenth revision, scheduled for publication in 2003, will use alphanumeric codes.

Joint Commission on the Accreditation of Healthcare Organizations A nonprofit organization that performs accreditation reviews primarily on hospitals, other institutional facilities, and outpatient facilities. Most managed care plans require any hospital under contract to be accredited by the Joint Commission.

lag study A report that tells managers how old the claims are that are being processed, how much is paid out each month (both for that month and for each earlier month), and how the amount paid out compares to the amount accrued for expenses. The lag study is a powerful tool for determining whether the plan's reserves are adequate to meet all expenses. Plans that fail to perform lag studies properly may find themselves staring into the abyss.

length of stay (LOS) The duration of a patient's stay in a hospital. An estimated length of stay is the duration a patient is expected to stay in a hospital based on the average length of stay from a large number of similar cases over time.

loss ratio *See* **medical loss ratio.**

managed care Also called *managed health care.* At the very least, managed care is a system of health care delivery that tries to control the cost of health care services while regulating access to those services and maintaining or improving their quality. A managed care organization typically has a panel of contracted providers that does not include all available providers, some type of limitations on benefits if subscribers use noncontracted providers (unless authorized to do so), and some type of authorization system. Managed care organizations range from preferred provider organizations to point-of-service plans, open-panel HMOs, and closed-panel HMOs.

managed care organization (MCO) An organization that delivers health care services using a managed care approach.

Some people prefer *managed care organization* to *health maintenance organization* because it encompasses plans that do not conform to the strict definition of an HMO (although that definition has loosened considerably). The term may also apply to a preferred provider organization, an exclusive provider organization, an integrated delivery system, or an OWA (other weird arrangement).

managed health care *See* **managed care.**

management information system (MIS) Computer hardware and software that helps manage the information necessary for running an organization.

management service organization (MSO) A type of integrated health delivery system. An MSO often purchases certain hard assets of a physician's practice and then provides services to the physician at fair market rates. MSOs are usually formed as a means to contract more effectively with managed care organizations, although their simple creation does not guarantee success. Some MSOs are similar to **service bureaus** (see below).

mandated benefits Benefits that a health plan is required by law to provide. Mandated benefits are generally benefits above and beyond routine insurance-type benefits, they are typically mandated by state laws, and the types of benefits mandated vary widely from state to state. Common examples include in vitro fertilization, defined days of inpatient mental health or substance abuse treatment, and other special-condition treatments. Self-funded plans are exempt from mandated benefits under ERISA.

mandatory external review A mandated review of a medical coverage decision by an unbiased external reviewer. The review of such decisions by a physician in an appropriate specialty has been mandated in some states and is widely undertaken on a voluntary basis in any event.

maximum allowable charge (MAC) The highest amount that a vendor may charge for something. The term is often used in pharmacy contracting. *Fee maximum* is a related term used in conjunction with professional fees.

maximum out-of-pocket cost The highest amount a member will ever need to pay for covered services during a contract year. The maximum out-of-pocket cost includes deductibles and coinsurance. Once this amount is reached, the health plan pays for all services up to the maximum level of coverage. Out-of-pocket cost limits are found mostly in non-HMO plans such as indemnity plans, preferred provider organizations, and point-of-service plans.

medical loss ratio The ratio between the cost of delivering medical care and the amount of money taken in by a plan. Insurance companies often have a medical loss ratio of 92 percent or more; tightly managed HMOs may have medical loss ratios of 75 to 85 percent, although the overhead (or administrative cost ratio) is concomitantly higher. The medical loss ratio is dependent on the amount of money brought in as well as the cost of delivering care; thus, if the rates are too low, the ratio may be high even though the cost of delivering care is not out of line.

medical policy The set of policies that a health plan uses to determine what medical services will be paid for and how much will be paid. Routine medical policy is linked to routine claims processing, which may even be automated. For example, a plan may only pay 50 percent of the fee of a second surgeon or may not pay for the second of two surgical procedures done during one episode of anesthesia. Medical policy also encompasses policies regarding payment for experimental or investigational care and for noncovered services in lieu of more expensive covered services.

medical savings account (MSA) A specialized savings account into which a consumer can put pretax dollars for use in paying medical expenses rather than purchase comprehensive health insurance or a managed care product. The user of an MSA must purchase a catastrophic health insurance policy as a "safety net" to protect against very high costs. MSAs were created as a demonstration under the Health Insurance Portability and Accountability Act and are currently known as *Archer MSAs*.

Medicare+Choice The revised form of the Medicare private insurance option. Medicare+Choice was created under the Balanced Budget Act of 1997.

Medigap insurance Health insurance that covers whatever Medicare does not. Medigap policies are now subject to minimum standards under federal law.

member An individual covered under a managed care plan. Members include subscribers and dependents.

member month One month of coverage for one member. For example, if a plan had 10,000 members in January and 12,000 members in February, the total member months for the year to date as of March 1 would be 22,000.

Mental Health Parity Act Act passed in 1996 that requires group health plans that offer mental health benefits to apply the same annual and aggregate lifetime dollar limits to the coverage of mental health services as those applied to the coverage of other services. The federal law applies to fully insured and self-insured plans, including state-regulated plans. However, states may enact requirements more stringent than those contained in the act.

midlevel practitioners (MLPs) Physician's assistants, clinical nurse practitioners, nurse midwives, and the like. Midlevel practitioners are nonphysicians who deliver medical care, generally under the supervision of a physician but for less cost.

Military Health System (MHS) A large and complex health care system designed to provide, and to maintain readiness to provide, medical services and support to the armed forces during military operations and to provide medical services and support to members of the armed forces, their dependents, and others entitled to Department of Defense (DoD) medical care. *See also* **CHAMPUS** and **TRICARE**.

mixed model A managed care plan that mixes two or more types of delivery systems. The term *mixed model* has traditionally been used to describe HMOs that have both closed-panel and open-panel delivery systems.

most favored nation discount A discount given by a provider to a payer based on a contractual agreement that stipulates the payer will automatically received the best discount given to anyone else.

National Association of Insurance Commissioners (NAIC) A voluntary national organization made up of the insurance commissioners from each state. The NAIC helps draft model legislation and regulations, but has no authority to impose such standards.

National Committee on Quality Assurance (NCQA) A nonprofit organization that performs quality-oriented accreditation reviews of HMOs and similar types of managed care plans. NCQA also accredits CVOs and develops HEDIS standards.

National Provider Identifier (NPI or NPID) A provider identifier mandated under the Health Insurance Portability and Accountability Act. The NPI will replace all other provider identifiers regardless of customer (i.e., commercial health plan, Medicare, Medicaid, CHAMPUS, and so forth). It is expected to be implemented in a rollout manner beginning in 2004. The NPI is proposed to be a 10-digit numeric identifier, with one of the digits being a checksum. It contains no embedded intelligence, such as information about the type of health care provider or the state where the health care provider is located. For the actual definition, which will be finalized after this book goes to press, visit www.hcfa.gov/stats/npi/overview.htm.

network model HMO A health plan that contracts with multiple physician groups, generally large single- or multispecialty groups, to deliver health care to members. Network model HMOs differ from group model plans, which contract with a single medical group; independent practice associations, which contract through an intermediary; and direct contract model plans, which contract with individual physicians in the community.

non-par Short for nonparticipating. The term refers to a provider that does not have a contract with the health plan.

Office of the Inspector General (OIG) The federal agency responsible for conducting investigations and audits of federal contractors or any system that receives funds or reimbursement from the federal government. There are OIG departments in different federal programs, including CHAMPUS, Medicare, and the Federal Employee Health Benefits Program.

Office of Managed Care (OMC) The federal agency that oversees federal qualification and compliance for HMOs and eligibility for CMPs. It was formerly called the Health Maintenance Organization Service, the Office of Health Maintenance Organizations, the Office of Prepaid Health Care, and the Office of Prepaid Health Care Operations and Oversight. Once part of the Public Health Service, OMC is now part of CMS. This agency could be reorganized yet again, and heaven only knows what its new acronym will be.

Office of Personnel Management (OPM) The federal agency that administers the **Federal Employee Health Benefits Program**. This is the agency with which a managed care plan contracts to provide coverage for federal employees.

open enrollment period The period when an employee may change health plans. It usually occurs once a year. A general rule is that a managed care plan will have around half its membership up for open enrollment in the fall for an effective date of January 1. A special type of open enrollment is mandated by law in some states. During this period an HMO must accept any individual applicant (i.e., not a member of an employer group) for coverage regardless of health status. Such special open enrollment periods usually last for one month and occur once a year. Many Blue Cross Blue Shield plans have similar open enrollment periods for indemnity products.

open-panel MCO A managed care plan that contracts (either directly or indirectly) with private physicians to deliver care in their own offices. Examples would include a direct contract HMO and an independent practice association.

other party liability (OPL) *See* **coordination of benefits.**

outlier Something that is well outside of an expected range. The term may refer to a provider who is using medical resources at a much higher rate than his or her peers or to a case in a hospital that is far more expensive than anticipated.

OWA (other weird arrangement) A general acronym that applies to any managed care plan with a new twist.

package pricing Also called *bundled pricing*. As an example, an MCO might pay an organization a single fee for all inpatient, outpatient, and professional expenses associated with a procedure, including preadmission and postdischarge care. This form of pricing is commonly used for cardiac bypass surgery and transplants.

par provider Shorthand term for participating provider (i.e., a provider who has signed an agreement with a plan to provide services). The term applies to professional and institutional providers.

peer review organization (PRO) An organization charged with reviewing quality and cost for Medicare. Established under the Tax Equity and Fiscal Responsibility Act, it generally operates at the state level.

pended claim A claim placed on hold. Although the terms *pend* and *suspend* are often used synonymously, some MCOs differentiate between claims placed on hold by examiners (pends) and claims placed on hold automatically by one or more system edits (suspends).

per diem reimbursement Reimbursement of an institution, usually a hospital, based on a set rate per day rather than on charges. Per diem reimbursement may vary by service (e.g., medical-surgical, obstetrics, mental health, and intensive care) or may be uniform regardless of the intensity of care.

per member per month (PMPM) Specifically applies to revenue or cost for each enrolled member each month.

per member per year (PMPY) The same as PMPM but based on a year.

per thousand members per year (PTMPY) A common way of reporting utilization. For instance, hospital utilization is commonly expressed as the number of hospital days per thousand members per year.

physician-hospital organization (PHO) A legal or informal organization that bonds a hospital and the attending medical staff. PHOs are frequently developed for the purpose of contracting with managed care plans. A PHO may be open to any member of the staff who applies or may be closed to staff members who fail to qualify (or whose specialty is already overrepresented).

physician incentive program A reimbursement methodology according to which a physician's income from an MCO (or an integrated delivery system) is affected by the physician's performance or by the overall performance of the organization (as measured by utilization, medical cost, quality measurements, member satisfaction, and so forth). As used by CMS, the term *physician incentive program* has a specific meaning. CMS limits the degree of incentive or risk allowed under a Medicare HMO (refer to the physician incentive program regulations at 42 C.F.R. 422.208/210 of the June 26, 1998, regulations that implement Medicare Part C), and it essentially bans "gainsharing" via a physician incentive program in an integrated delivery system receiving reimbursement under Medicare. Some states also now have laws and regulations that place limits on physician incentive programs and require the disclosure of physician incentives to members enrolled in MCOs. *See also* **significant financial risk**.

physician practice management company (PPMC) A company that manages physician practices and in most cases either owns the practices outright or has the right to purchase them in the future. PPMCs concentrate only on physicians and not on hospitals, although some PPMCs have also entered into joint ventures with hospitals and insurers. Many PPMCs are publicly traded.

PlanID Identifier mandated under the Health Insurance Portability and Accountability Act. The PlanID will be the identifier used by health plans (broadly defined) when conducting all transactions. The PlanID will be affected by the benefits design. The PlanID is expected to be implemented in a rollout fashion beginning in 2004.

point-of-service (POS) plan A plan where members do not have to choose how to receive services until they need them. The term commonly applies to a plan that enrolls each member in both an HMO (or HMO-like system) and an indemnity plan. This type of plan is occasionally referred to as an *HMO swingout plan,* an *out-of-plan benefits rider to an HMO,* or a *primary care preferred provider organization.* In a point-of-service plan, the coverage differs depending on whether the member chooses to use the plan's providers (e.g., 100-percent coverage) or go outside the plan for services (e.g., 70-percent coverage). A dual choice plan encompasses an HMO-like plan and an indemnity plan, and a triple choice plan adds a preferred provider organization to the mix. Although this usage is archaic, the term *point-of-service plan* can refer to a simple preferred provider organization, where members receive a higher level of coverage if they use preferred providers.

precertification Also called *preadmission certification, preadmission review,* and *precert.* Precertification is the process of obtaining certification or authorization from a health plan for routine medical services (inpatient or outpatient). Precertification often involves an appropriateness review and the assignment of a length of stay. Failure to obtain precertification typically results in a financial penalty to either the provider or the subscriber.

preexisting condition A medical condition for which a member has received treatment during a specified period of time prior to becoming covered under a health plan. Treatment for preexisting conditions may not be covered by certain types of health plans.

preferred provider organization (PPO) A plan that contracts with independent providers at a discount for services. The panel is limited in size and usually has some type of utilization review system associated with it. A PPO may be risk bearing, like an insurance company, or non-risk-bearing, like a physician-sponsored PPO that markets itself to insurance companies or self-insured companies.

premium equivalent Calculated amount used by a self-insured employer to determine its own costs, necessary payroll deductions, and so forth. The premium equivalent is equal to what the premium rate have would to be if the self-insured employer were an insured benefits plan. An MCO may count premium equivalent along with actual premium for purposes of calculating medical costs, administrative costs, and so forth, since the costs are independent of where the final risk for those costs resides.

premium rate The rate that an MCO charges its customers for health benefits coverage. For example, the premium rate may be $500 per employee per month, which is what the MCO bills the employer. The employer may deduct some part of that from each employee's paycheck and then send the total amount of money to the MCO.

preventive care Health care that is aimed at preventing complications of existing diseases or preventing the occurrence of diseases.

primary care physician (PCP) Generally applies to internists, pediatricians, family physicians, and general practitioners and occasionally to Ob/Gyns.

prospective payment system (PPS) A system for determining fixed pricing for reimbursement of hospitals and other health care facilities. The best-known PPS is the classification system consisting of diagnostic-related groups, but the ambulatory patient classification system is another example.

prospective review Reviewing the need for medical care before the care is rendered. *See also* **precertification.**

protected health information (PHI) Medical information that is individually identifiable; in other words, a combination of medical information and some other data that links that medical information to an individual. The issue of protected health information is addressed by the Health Insurance Portability and Accountability Act in the Privacy and Security sections.

provider Any person or organization that provides medical services. The term is most often used to refer to physicians. How physicians went from being called *physicians* to being called *providers* is unclear, although it probably has to do with the fact that other types of health care professionals, such as physician assistants and nurse practitioners, also provide primary care. In any case, although the use of *provider* is not embraced by physicians, the term is used widely, including in this book.

provider-sponsored organization (PSO) A risk-bearing managed care organization made up of providers that contracts directly with the Health Care Financing Administration for Medicare enrollees. The rules for financial solvency for PSOs are somewhat different than for HMOs, and if a PSO is not licensed by the state, it can seek licensure directly from the Health Care Financing Administration. PSOs came about because providers and legislators thought that there were fat profits to be had by "cutting out the middle man"—that is, removing HMOs from the equation. A few PSOs actually got started under a demonstration program, and a few more came into being under the Balance Budget Act of 1997. Most failed utterly, though a few remain.

prudent layperson standard *See* **reasonable layperson standard.**

quality assurance (QA) *See* **quality management**.

Quality Improvement System for Managed Care (QISMC) A CMS initiative designed to strengthen the efforts of MCOs to protect and improve the health and satisfaction of Medicare and Medicaid beneficiaries. QISMC, using a very broad definition of quality, focuses on "measurement of health outcomes, consumer satisfaction, the accountability of managed care organizations for achieving ongoing quality improvement, the need for intervention to achieve this improvement, and the importance of data collection, analysis, and reporting."

quality management (QM) Refers to the tools and techniques used by an MCO or a provider to ensure that the quality of health care delivery is acceptable. Most programs go further, and look for ways to continually improve quality of health care delivery.

rate The amount of money that a group or an individual must pay to a health plan for coverage. The payment is usually in the form of a monthly fee. The term *rating* refers to the development of rates by a health plan.

reasonable layperson standard A standard applied in determining whether medical care is warranted and also whether a health plan should provide payment for medical care given. The standard is almost always invoked in cases where a patient could possibly be viewed as needing emergency or urgent care. Even though a trained provider may not think that urgent care is required, if a reasonable layperson has good reason to believe that such care should be provided, the standard entails that so it should. In regards to Medicare and Medicaid enrollees, the specific language used in the Balanced Budget Act of 1997 is as follows: "Health plans should provide payment when a consumer presents to an emergency department with acute symptoms of sufficient severity—including severe pain—such that a 'prudent layperson' could reasonably expect the absence of medical attention to result in placing health in serious jeopardy, serious impairment to bodily functions, or serious dysfunction of any bodily organ or part."

reinsurance Insurance purchased by a health plan to protect it against extremely high-cost cases. *See also* **stop-loss insurance.**

relative value unit (RVU) A number used as a multiplier in order to calculate the payment to a provider. In an RVU system, a value is assigned to each procedure or visit code, and the fee is determined by multiplying the value by a set dollar amount. For example, if a procedure had a relative value of 4.5 and the set amount was $10, the fee for the procedure would be $45. Not consistent or uniform, RVUs are often based on national standards but altered as a result of negotiation. *See also* **resource-based relative value scale.**

reserves The amount of money that a health plan puts aside to cover health care costs. The reserves may include money the plan keeps as a cushion against unexpectedly high future health care costs.

resource-based relative value scale (RBRVS) A relative value scale developed for the Health Care Financing Administration (CMS) for use by Medicare. The RBRVS assigns a relative value to each CPT code on the basis of the resources related to the procedure rather than simply on the basis of historical trends. The practical effect has been to lower reimbursement for procedural services (e.g., cardiac surgery) and to raise reimbursement for cognitive services (e.g., office visits).

retrospective review Reviewing health care costs after the care has been rendered. There are two types of retrospective review. One looks at individual claims to assess medical necessity and discover billing errors or fraud; the other looks at patterns of cost rather than individual cases.

risk-based capital (RBC) A formula embodied in the Risk-Based Capital for Health Organizations Model Act, created under the auspices of the National Association of Insurance Commissioners. RBC takes into account the fluctuating value of plan assets, the financial condition of plan affiliates, the risk that providers may not be able to provide contracted services, the risk that amounts due may not be recovered from reinsurance carriers, and general business risk (i.e., the risk that expenses may exceed income). The RBC formula gives credit for provider payment arrangements that reduce underwriting risk, including capitation, provider withholds, bonuses, contracted fee schedules, and aggregate cost arrangements. While only required in a handful of states and collected in approximately 40 states (as of 2000), RBC is the agreed standard to be used by an insurance department in determining whether a health plan meets minimum financial solvency requirements. Under the provisions of the act (whose adoption by each state is voluntary), if a plan's total capital assets fall below 200 percent of the risk-based capital requirement, state regulators may require the plan to submit its own proposal for corrective action. If total capital assets fall below 150 percent of the capital requirement, regulators may perform their own analysis and issue a corrective order defining necessary actions to solve the problem. If total capital assets fall below 100 percent of the capital requirement, the state may place the plan under "regulatory control," and if the level falls below 70 percent, the state is required to do so.

risk contract Also known as a *Medicare risk contract.* A contract between an HMO or CMP and CMS to provide services to Medicare beneficiaries in return for a fixed monthly payment for each enrolled Medicare member.

risk management Management activities aimed at lowering an organization's legal and financial exposure, especially to lawsuits.

SCHIP *See* **Children's Health Insurance Program.**

second opinion An opinion obtained from another physician regarding the necessity for a treatment that has been recommended by the first physician. A second opinion is required by some health plans for certain high-cost treatments or operations, such as cardiac surgery.

self-insured plan Also called a *self-funded plan.* In a self-insured plan, the risk for medical cost is assumed by the employer rather than an insurance company or managed care plan. Under the Employee Retirement Income Security Act, self-insured plans are exempt from state laws and regulations and from paying premium taxes. Self-insured plans often contract with insurance companies or third-party administrators to administer the benefits. *See also* **administrative services only (ASO) contract**.

service area The geographic area in which an MCO provides access to primary care. The service area is usually specifically designated by the regulators (state or federal), and the MCO is prohibited from marketing outside of the service area. The service area may be defined by county or ZIP code boundaries. It is possible for an MCO to have more than one service area and for the service areas to be contiguous or noncontiguous.

service bureau A weak form of integrated delivery system in which a hospital (or other organization) provides services to a physician's practice in return for a fair market price. The service bureau may also try to negotiate with managed care plans, but it is generally not considered to be an effective negotiating mechanism.

service plan A health insurance plan that has direct contract with providers but is not necessarily a managed care plan. The archetypal service plans are Blue Cross and Blue Shield plans, and these are virtually the only plans that fall into this category. The contract applies to direct billing of the plan by providers (rather than billing of the members), contains a provision for direct payment of the providers (rather than reimbursement of the members), requires that the providers accept the plan's determination of usual, customary, or reasonable fees and not balance-bill the members in excess of these amounts, and has a range of other provisions. The contract may or may not address utilization and quality issues.

shock claim Also referred to as a *catastrophic claim.* A shock claim is a claim with an extraordinarily high total cost. Shock claims are taken into account by actuaries when they determine medical cost trends, although these claims tend to appear randomly and infrequently.

significant financial risk (SFR) A substantial risk of income loss. The term *financial risk* is used by CMS to refer to the total amount of a physician's income at risk in a Medicare HMO. Such financial risk is considered "significant" when it exceeds a certain percentage of the total potential income that the physician could receive under the reimbursement program. According to a common definition, any physician incentive payment program that allows for a variation of more than 25 percent between the minimum and the maximum amount of potential reimbursement would place the physicians at significant financial risk.

specialty care physician A physician who is not a primary care provider.

staff model HMO An HMO in which providers are directly employed by the organization and see members in the organization's own facilities (in other words, a type of closed-panel HMO). The term is also sometimes applied to vertically integrated health care delivery systems that employ physicians but are not licensed as HMOs.

Stark regulations Regulations named after "Pete" Fortney Stark, congressman from California. The so-called Stark regulations are actually two sets of regulations: Stark I and Stark II. These regulations are not for amateurs to handle. Indeed, competent legal counsel is required for any provider system doing business with federal or state governments.

state of domicile The state in which an insurance company or MCO is licensed as its primary location. For example, the state of domicile for an MCO may be Virginia, but the MCO might also be licensed and doing business in Maryland and the District of Columbia. In many states, the insurance commissioner will defer primary regulation to the insurance department in the state of domicile as long as all minimum standards of the state are met.

stop-loss insurance A form of reinsurance that provides protection against medical expenses above a certain limit, generally on a year-by-year basis. Stop-loss insurance may apply to an entire health plan or to any single component. For example, the health plan may have stop-loss insurance for cases that exceed $100,000. After a case hits $100,000, the plan receives 80 percent of expenses in excess of $100,000 from the reinsurance company for the rest of the year. In another example, a plan might provide a form of stop-loss insurance to participating physicians for referral expenses over $2,500. If a case exceeds that amount in a single year, the plan would no longer deduct the costs from the physician's referral pool for the remainder of the year. Specific coverage pertains to individual high-cost cases, while aggregate coverage pertains to the total costs.

subrogation The contractual right of a health plan to recover payments made to a member for health care costs after that member has received such payments for damages in a legal action. In other words, if a person is injured in an auto accident and sues the other driver for damages, part of the calculation of damages included medical costs. The MCO has the right to collect that amount of the damage award (if there is one) since it paid the medical costs already. Subrogation is not allowed in all states.

subscriber The individual or member who has the health plan coverage in virtue of being eligible on his or her own behalf rather than as a dependent.

Sutton's law Go where the money is! Attributed to the Depression-era bank robber Willy Sutton, who, when asked why he robbed banks, replied, "That's where the money is." Sutton apparently denies ever having made that statement. In any event, it is a good law to use when determining what needs attention in a managed care plan.

Tax Equity and Fiscal Responsibility Act (TEFRA) An act that prohibits employers and health plans from requiring full-time employees between the ages of 65 and 69 to use Medicare rather than the group health plan. Another key provision codifies Medicare risk contracts for HMOs and CMPs.

Temporary Assistance to Needy Families (TANF) A federal program that provides Medicaid to families that meet low-income criteria and in which mothers and children require medical assistance.

termination date The day that health plan coverage ceases to be in effect.

third-party administrator (TPA) A firm that performs administrative functions (e.g., claims processing, membership services, and the like) for a self-funded plan or a start-up managed care plan. *See also* **administrative services only (ASO) contract.**

total capitation *See* **global capitation.**

triage Originally, the process of sorting out wounded soldiers into those who need treatment immediately, those who can wait, and those who are too severely injured to even try to save. In health plans, *triage* refers to the process of sorting out requests for services by members into those who need to be seen right away, those who can wait a little while, and those whose problems can be handled over the phone.

TRICARE The Department of Defense's worldwide managed health care program. TRICARE was initiated in 1995, integrating health care services provided in the direct care system of military hospitals and clinics with services purchased under CHAMPUS. *See also* **Civilian Health and Medical Program of the Uniformed Services** and **military health system.**

turn-around time (TAT) The amount of time it takes a health plan to process and pay a claim after it arrives.

UB-92 The common claim form used by hospitals to bill for services. Some managed care plans demand greater detail than is available on the UB-92, requiring the hospitals to send additional itemized bills. Because of the passage of the Health Insurance Portability and Accountability Act, this form will be used infrequently in the future, since it is not the same as the electronic format required under the act's final rule for transactions.

unbundling The practice of billing for multiple components of a medical procedure or service that were previously included in a single fee. For example, in a case where dressings and instruments had been included in a fee for a minor procedure, unbundling would involve charging a fee for the procedure itself (perhaps a fee of the same amount) and additional fees for the dressings and instruments.

underwriting Bearing the risk for something (e.g., a policy is underwritten by an insurance company). The term can also be used to refer to (1) analyzing a group to determine rates and benefits or whether the group should be offered coverage at all and (2) health screening each individual applicant for insurance, and basing the type of coverage and the cost of such coverage on the results of that screening.

Universal Provider Identification (UPIN) An identification number issued by the Health Care Financing Administration for use in billing Medicare. The UPIN will be replaced by the National Provider Identifier (NPI) some time in 2004; in fact, all provider identification numbers will be replaced by the NPI.

upcoding The practice of a billing for a procedure that pays better than the procedure actually performed. For example, an office visit that would normally be reimbursed at $45 is coded as one that is reimbursed at $53.

U.S. Department of Health and Human Services (DHHS) Cabinet-level federal department that oversees many programs, including the Centers for Medicare & Medicaid Services, which is responsible for Medicare and Medicaid (in conjunction with individual states). The department also has oversight responsibility for the **Health Insurance Portability and Accountability Act** and related federal legislation.

U.S. Department of Labor Federal department that regulates coverage offered to employees when an employer retains the insurance risk (i.e., self-funding pursuant to ERISA) either on a stand-alone basis or through a multiple employer welfare arrangement.

usual, customary, or reasonable (UCR) Profiling prevailing fees in an area and reimbursing providers on the basis of the resulting profile. One archaic method is to average all fees and choose the 80th or 90th percentile, although in this era a plan will usually use another method to determine what is reasonable. Sometimes *usual, customary, or reasonable* is used to refer to a fee allowance schedule when the schedule is set relatively high.

Utilization Review Accreditation Commission (URAC) A nonprofit organization that performs reviews of external utilization review agencies (freestanding companies, utilization management departments of insurance companies, and utilization management departments of managed care plans). Its primary focus is managed indemnity and preferred provider organizations, though it has expanded its accreditation activities. States often require certification by URAC for a utilization management organization to operate. URAC is also known as the American Accreditation Healthcare Commission (AAHC).

utilization review organization (URO) A freestanding organization that does nothing but utilization review, usually on a remote basis, using the telephone and paper correspondence.

It may be independent or part of another company, such as an insurance company that sells utilization review services on a stand-alone basis.

workers' compensation A form of social insurance provided through property-casualty insurers. Workers' compensation provides medical benefits and replacement of lost wages that result from injuries or illnesses that occur in the workplace; in turn, an injured or sick employee cannot normally sue the employer unless true negligence exists. Because workers' compensation has undergone dramatic increases in cost recently, workers' compensation carriers are now adopting managed care approaches. Workers' compensation is often heavily regulated under state laws that are significantly different than those that pertain to group health insurance, and workers' compensation provisions are often the subject of intense negotiation between management and organized labor.

wraparound plan Insurance or health plan coverage for co-pays and deductibles that exist as part of a member's base plan. Wraparound plans are often used for Medicare.

zero down The practice of distributing all of a group's capital surplus to the members of the group rather than retaining any capital or reinvesting it.

Index

A

Access, 127–128
  Health Insurance Portability and Accountability Act, 225–227
  managed care organization, 104–105
  Medicare+Choice, standards, 206–207
Accreditation, managed care organization, 239–240
  accreditation organizations, 239–240
Accrete, 259
Accrual, 259
Accrued revenue, 186
Actuarial assumptions, 259
Actuarial services, 190
Adjusted average per capita cost, 259–260
Adjusted community rate, 260

Adjusted community rating, 191, 266
Administration of benefits, 170–173
Administrative costs, finance department, 188
Administrative services, 157–158
Administrative services only (ASO) contract, 260
Administrative simplification, Health Insurance Portability and Accountability Act, 228–236
  code sets, 229–232
  national identifier, 233
  privacy, 233
  security, 235–236
  transactions, 229–232
Adverse selection, 260
Alternative delivery system, 26
Amara's Law, 260–261

Q